2-10

MIXED
SIGNALS

MIXED
SIGNALS

Understanding and Treating Your Child's Sensory Processing Issues

Mary Lashno, O.T.

Woodbine House ◆ 2010

All rights reserved under International and Pan-American copyright conventions.
Published in the United States of America by Woodbine House, Inc., 6510 Bells Mill
Road, Bethesda, MD 20817. 800-843-7323. www.woodbinehouse.com

Library of Congress Cataloging-in-Publication Data

Lashno, Mary.
  Mixed signals : understanding and treating your child's sensory processing issues /
by Mary Lashno. -- 1st ed.
      p. cm.
  Includes bibliographical references and index.
  ISBN 978-1-890627-59-1
  1. Sensory integration dysfunction in children--Popular works. I. Title.
  RJ496.S44.L37 2009
  618.92'8--dc22

                                                              2009034621

Manufactured in the United States of America

First Edition

10   9   8   7   6   5   4   3   2   1

To my husband, Walt, and my family for all the encouragement and support they have given me while writing this book. Mostly, I thank my son, Michael, who introduced me to the world of autism and allowed me to explore his strategies for learning to cope and live in his world of mixed signals.

Table of Contents

1 What is Sensory Processing?

The Jones Family

Emma and Allison are the young children of Mrs. Jones. Emma is a typically developing two-year-old who loves to sit on her mother's lap and listen to soft lullabies. As her mother touches her arm, Emma looks up at her and smiles. Information from touch and hearing are processed in Emma's brain and are perceived as a pleasant experience. Emma reaches out to get a hug and begins to sing along to the music.

When Allison, Emma's five-year-old sister, is encouraged to join in, she responds in a completely different fashion. Allison refuses to sit on her mother's lap and as her mother tries to reach out to cuddle her, she reacts by screaming and running away. Allison is also processing the above-mentioned information, but she perceives the singing and touch as a danger—something to avoid. Allison's negative reaction does not reflect her feelings for her mother; rather, her brain is simply unable to understand and process the information needed for her to perceive this as a pleasant experience. The result is that Mrs. Jones must put Emma down on the floor so she can try to calm Allison. Saddened by the loss of attention, Emma begins to cry and as she does, Allison places her hands over her ears and runs towards Emma. She pushes her roughly and Emma falls to the floor, causing her to cry even louder.

Mrs. Jones becomes upset with Allison, but the more she tries to reason with her (while Emma continues to cry) the more Allison screams and lashes out. Mrs. Jones ends up taking Allison to her room so she can "think about what she has done." Her room is quiet and dark, and once *alone, Allison crawls up on her bed and nestles under a heavy blanket, quietly humming one of the lullabies to herself until she falls asleep.*

This story illustrates the difference between a sensory processing system that is operating properly—Emma's—and one that isn't—Allison's. Sensory processing is the neurological process of our nervous system to take information from our body or the environment, organize it in the brain, and determine the correct behavioral or physiological response to the various types of input. For someone with no sensory integration weaknesses, this feedback loop happens naturally and quickly. Input comes from all of our senses: sight, hearing, taste, touch, smell, body position, and movement.

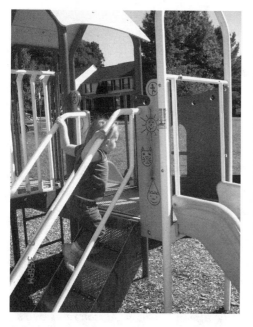

Sensory processing is the cornerstone for the development of all motor and social skills, and enables us to learn and engage in higher level tasks, such as playing on the playground, self-feeding, participating in dressing, and academic pursuits, to name a few.

Unfortunately, people with poor sensory processing systems are unable to "make sense" of environmental information and may display odd behaviors in response to sensory input. (Some typically seen behaviors are listed in the section below.) This condition is known as Sensory Processing Disorder (SPD). It is also sometimes referred to as Sensory (Integration) Dysfunction (SID) or Sensory Modulation Disorder (SMD). Illustrated by the story of Allison, you can easily imagine how sensory processing problems can affect the bond between a mother and child, and how, if this behavior is demonstrated with all types of sensory input, it can affect the relationship the child has with the entire family, his schoolmates and teachers, and the larger community.

Does This Sound Like Your Child?

Below is a list of some of the behaviors you may observe in your child that may result from sensory processing problems. You may notice that some of these behaviors seem contradictory, i.e., "avoids touching objects" and "touches everything." This is because people with SPD can have over-reactions or under-reactions to sensory input. Interestingly, a person with SPD doesn't always react to stimuli in a predictable manner; for example, they might respond in an over-exaggerated way to the sound of a vacuum or blender by screaming and running away, but might under-react to the sound of a blaring fire alarm just outside the room. Typical behaviors exhibited by a child with a sensory processing disorder may include:

- Does not enjoy "fun" events or group gatherings, rather tends to scream and cry, run away and hide in a dark, quiet space;
- Does not really use his hands, avoids touching objects or certain textures, holding utensils, putting hands in sandbox, etc;
- Only wants to wear certain clothing, usually old worn-out or well-washed clothing;
- Hates to have face washed, teeth brushed, hair combed or cut;
- Touches everything;
- Holds ears or overreacts to "everyday" noises;
- Stares at lights;
- Runs around a room and appears overwhelmed, especially in a mall or visually stimulating environment (birthday party, preschool setting);
- Does not actively engage in activities, tends to be more of an observer;
- Will not try new foods and is considered a "picky" eater;
- Stuffs mouth with food or is always chewing on nonedible objects;
- Seems unaware of where he is in his environment, bumps into walls, trips over toys, seems overly clumsy;
- Seems overly rough with toys and people (doesn't seem to know his own strength);
- Physically lashes out at others;

- Becomes upset if his routine is changed;
- Engages in self-stimulatory or perseverative behaviors, such as rocking, flicking fingers, head-banging, etc.

Many children who have a sensory processing disorder will exhibit "strange behaviors" such as the examples given above. (Keep in mind, however, that depending on a child's age, some of these behaviors might be developmentally appropriate for a typically developing child or one with ASD without a sensory processing disorder.) A possible explanation is that even though a child is unable to process sensory information effectively, the brain still demands a response to sensory information. Many children need to seek out sensory input, such as flapping, or rapidly moving a hand in front of a light source. This may seem weird to us, but it is actually an attempt to provide "seeing and touching" information to the brain. Although abnormal, it is a way to try to make sense of the world. Unfortunately, it is not functional and because some children with sensory processing problems become obsessed with this type of stimulus, they often refuse to participate in "normal" activities. Many families, when they witness their child engaging in these types of behaviors, are overwhelmed, fearful, and overflowing with questions. You may worry: Is my kid doing these things deliberately? Is it a matter of not disciplining him enough? Will he outgrow these behaviors? What makes him act this way and why doesn't he "fit in"? You may wonder: Why does our child have such difficulty with sensory processing and how do we help him overcome these issues so he can be an integrated member of our family? Although the behaviors of children with a sensory processing disorder may often seem strange to us, they are actually valiant—albeit abnormal—attempts to make sense of the world. (See Chapter 4 for more in depth information on the diagnostic process.)

Sensory Processing and Autism Spectrum Disorders

Most children with autism spectrum disorders (ASD) share a cluster of characteristics, including impairments in social skills, communication, and ritualistic, repetitive activities and interests. These symptoms can reveal themselves as poor social and play skills, difficulty using speech and understanding verbal directions, problems with transitioning from one activity to another, odd behaviors, and more. In addition to these traits, children with ASD also have difficulty processing sensory information and many exhibit the types of "odd" behaviors listed in the earlier section.

Although the Diagnostic and Statistical Manual of Mental Disorders–IV (DMS-IV) does not currently include poor sensory processing as part of the diagnostic criteria for an autism spectrum disorder (ASD), research continues to demonstrate that people with ASD tend to have many more issues with sensory processing than the general population (Kientz & Dunn, 1997; Watling, Deitz & White, 2001). Information that has been gathered from parents of typically developing children, children with developmental disabilities, and those with ASD shows that those with ASD demonstrate sensory symptoms specifically identified in taste, smell, tactile (touch), and auditory (hearing) processing (Rogers, Hepburn & Wehner, 2003). This growing body of research suggests that people with ASD often over- or under-process sensory input from the environment (Ornitz, 1989; Wainwright-Sharp and Bryson, 1993) or have trouble regulating sensory information (Lincoln et. al., 1993, 1995). Although ASD is an umbrella term and describes people who are affected across a broad continuum, sensory processing problems don't discriminate and are seen in people diagnosed with Asperger's disorder as well as those more severely affected by classic autism.

If your child has been diagnosed with ASD and he engages in many of the quirky behaviors listed above, it's challenging to tease out which of these behaviors are caused by autism and which are caused by sensory processing problems. Those caused by ASD can be dealt with using the many reputable behavior management techniques in practice today, and those identified as specifically sensory issues can be controlled through the use of sensory strategies. It may not be necessary to determine which behaviors are caused by what source, but simply *that* some of your child's odd behaviors are caused by sensory processing problems and are not all "just autism." In fact, research from as early as 1974 (Ornitz) hypothesized that abnormal sensory modulation was a primary symptom in autism, resulting in poor communication skills and a decreased ability to relate socially. This is not to say that children with autism will demonstrate odd behaviors as a result of their diagnosis of autism, but it is conceivable to think that through use of a sensory diet, some of their odd behaviors can be extinguished by providing the adequate amount of sensory input.

Strategies that provide the child with deep pressure, swinging, and vibration (all of which will be described later in detail), as part of a sensory diet may enable a child's dysfunctional sensory system to accept adequate input (for example, holding objects in hand, tolerating sitting in a circle with other children, etc.) The purpose of this book is to provide various strategies and practical information that will allow the child with ASD and/or sensory processing problems, along with help from his family, teachers, and school specialists (occupational therapists, speech-language therapists, behavioral therapists, aides, and psychologists), to adapt to the demands of everyday activities. A sensory diet can be used by a child anywhere on the autism spectrum, from those with Asperger's disorder to those most severely affected.

What are Sensory Strategies?

Although these will be discussed in detail in Chapter 7, this may be a good time to at least introduce some sensory strategies to give you a sense of what sensory integration therapy is all about. As stated earlier, a child with sensory processing disorder (SPD) is constantly being bombarded with sensory information. Depending on how that child's sensory system is functioning, the information may be viewed as "too much" or "too little." The goal of a sensory based approach is to help provide the "just right" amount of input in order to help the child regulate his sensory system and adapt to improve attention and focus for learning to occur. Below are brief descriptions of some of the sensory strategies that are used in treatment sessions and would be incorporated into a child's sensory diet for home and school.

A Sensory Diet

The term "sensory diet" has nothing to do with food but rather is a planned and scheduled activity program designed to meet a child's specific sensory needs. The "diet" of sensory information will consist of strategies that will enable the child to either "calm down" or "wake up" his sensory system, in order for learning to take place. These specific sensory strategies are provided at certain, established times of the day, and on an as-needed basis. A sensory diet is usually developed by an Occupational Therapist (OT), who has been trained in the use of various sensory approaches. She will typically observe the child and interview the child's family. Various types of sensory input will be tried with constant attention paid to the child's response to the input.

Sensory strategies might include **movement activities,** such as swinging, rocking, jumping, or rolling. This type of input stimulates the vestibular system and depending on how and when it is used, can either calm or alert the child. **Deep pressure** to the muscles and joints underlying the skin or heavy **touch pressure** to the skin receptors are calming types of input and can help the child regulate his sensory system and ready it for new input. **Proprioception**, or sensation to the joints and muscles, allows the child to begin to know where his body is in relation to space. Proprioceptive activities can either calm or alert a child and include jumping, playing tug of war, doing push-ups, or any type of activity that has the arms or legs pushing or pulling to activate the compression or contraction of the muscles and joints. **Joint compression** involves the delivery of a quick jolt of sensory input to a child's joint (e.g., elbow). A therapist or trained individual places her hands above and below the joint and compresses. This sends information to the child's brain which releases proprioceptive input, which can be calming or alerting. The use of **sensory tools** helps a child alert or calm to sensory input. Examples of these are soft surgical **brushes** that are used to apply deep, firm pressure to the arms and legs, and **vibrating toys** that can also calm or alert a child, depending on a child's needs. **Music** may also be used—either soft and rhythmic, which has a calming effect, or loud with changing tempos, which serves to alert a child.

Children may initially be upset by these techniques but usually become more agreeable to them over time and greater exposure, and will gradually increase their tolerance to various forms of sensory input. These activities and techniques will be further explained in a way that will make them simple to use on a daily basis. Keep in mind, however, that this book is not meant to take the place of guidance and advice from a trained and licensed occupational therapist.

Is the Sensory Based Approach Safe?

You may wonder what type of evidence or research supports this therapy as a viable approach. Currently, the research is limited, but

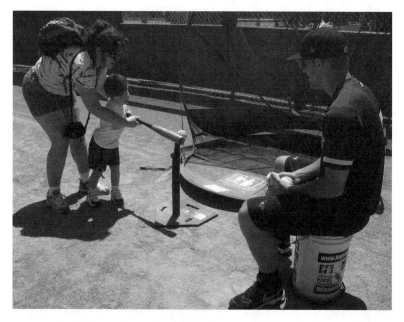

many research projects are being developed and data are being collected to support the efficacy of using a sensory based approach. In my own clinical experience, I have observed children overcoming all kinds of sensory defensiveness by using these techniques. For example, kids who initially refused to hold objects, choosing instead to mouth them, have gone on to use their hands to explore and use toys more appropriately. And kids who initially gagged on the texture of cracker crumbs mixed in baby food have learned to love hamburgers! I have had the pleasure of working with many parents frustrated with their child's behavior and eager for my advice. These strategies have done wonders to engage their children in play or help them to calm, along with increasing their ability to engage in daily activities and learning.

Using various sensory strategies and a sensory diet is sometimes a direct but noninvasive approach to addressing sensory issues in children. Positive or negative results are gauged by observing your child's body language, along with his ability to show increased interest in formally aversive objects or activities. The only real danger from this type of therapy would result from not understanding or respecting your child's initial response to the input. Although most children will learn to build up a tolerance for formally aversive types of input, it must be done slowly and at the "just right" level of tolerance for that particular child. If the stimulus continues to be forced and the child is screaming, then he is unable to process it and just wants you to stop. These issues and more will be explained in greater detail throughout this book.

Currently, there is no cure for ASD and use of a sensory based approach should not be viewed as a potential cure. This type of therapy will help your child feel more comfortable with sensory input and through use of the various strategies should allow your child to begin to tolerate input and increase his interaction both with objects and his environment.

Can This Book Help My Child or Student?

Depending of your child's specific diagnosis and unique set of skills and deficits, you may wonder if this book is appropriate for you and your family. Rest assured, the information covered in this book will be useful for all children on the autism spectrum, from those that display the full range of ASD symptoms, including those who are non-verbal and have limited interactions with people or objects, and those that are less severely affected by ASD. Whether a child is sitting in a corner and flicking his fingers in front of his face or chewing bits of paper when in an anxiety-provoking situation, once sensory-related behaviors are identified, there is a good chance that sensory input can be used in a positive manner to help calm or alert those children for participation in life's activities.

You may recognize your child or student in the case studies sprinkled throughout this book. They're intended to help you understand how a sensory processing disorder can affect your child's ability to participate in daily activities, such as play, interacting with family and friends, performing everyday tasks (self-feeding, dressing, etc.), and educational pursuits. In other words, this book will provide information as to how abnormal sensory processing will affect a child's ability to learn from his world. These are important concerns and ones that will be addressed in depth in this book. Without intervention, many of these abnormal attempts to make sense of sensory input will turn into established, inappropriate behaviors and will not only become part of a person's daily routine but will also become more difficult to extinguish as time goes on.

The ultimate goal for this book is to explain sensory processing and shed light onto why your child does these funny things with his body. Equally important, I'd like to provide families with strategies that may help them increase their child's ability to tolerate sensory input and enable their child to be a more active participant within the family unit, exhibit more appropriate behavior, become safer and more calmed, and able to attend and learn.

This book will also help both teacher and therapist to gather the appropriate information about her student and amply justify to the school that before it can ask a child with sensory issues to hold a pencil or sit in a circle, it first needs to help that child to calm or alert his sensory system in order to "get ready" to learn. Teachers justifiably feel confused and frustrated about how to meet the needs of the many kids in their classrooms with ASD and sensory processing issues. Teaching a child with ASD is challenge enough, but add a sensory processing disorder (SPD) on top of that and even the most seasoned teacher can become overwhelmed.

School therapists may also feel overwhelmed when they are called in to help a child with SPD but are not quite sure how to provide the types of therapy he may need. This book will introduce both teachers and therapists to the use of various techniques (e.g., brushing, deep pressure) along with providing recommendations for setting up a supportive environment (i.e., a quiet "chill out" area for a child who is having difficulty calming down). It will also provide information that will enable teachers and school therapists to recognize specific sensory-related behaviors that a child may be exhibiting and what type of sensory input he might be seeking. For example, a child pushing and hitting other children at circle time may need to sit in a beanbag chair, providing "deep pressure" to satisfy his over-responsive sensory system.

Throughout the book, case studies will illustrate the many different types of behaviors affected by a child's inability to appropriately process sensory information. This will allow us to more easily break down and tackle the ways sensory integration therapy can be used to positively affect these behaviors. Your child may not mimic the symptoms of any one particular child we describe, but you may notice surprising similarities across several of them. If so, rest assured you've made the right decision to pick up this book. You're well on you way to learning strategies that will help eradicate some of your child's odd or seemingly senseless behaviors and improve his participation as an active student or family member.

About this Book

Throughout this book, I will use male pronouns to refer to all children with sensory processing disorder (SPD) and female pronouns for all references to occupational therapists (OT) and teachers. In the early chapters of this book I will breakdown terminology related to sensory 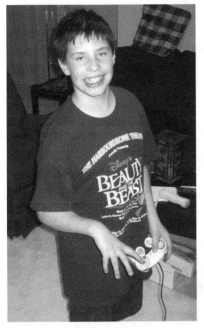 processing and explain why sensory processing is important to our ability to learn and function within our environment. I will contrast a child with a normal sensory processing system and a child who is experiencing an abnormal sensory system. I'll then describe the various sensory behaviors often present in a child with ASD and how they affect the child's ability to make sense of his world. Even though many of these behaviors seem strange to us, they may possibly be a child with ASD's way of adapting to his environment. I'll provide some possible rationales for why your child or student is acting a certain way in specific situations and provide information about the diagnostic/evaluation process. The second half of this book will discuss various treatment approaches, and goals and expectations of therapy. The last section of the book will provide practical solutions that may help your child both at home and school.

I intend for this book to validate your concerns as parents and help you become more astute in understanding both your child's behavior and possible ways to encourage a "more normal" response to sensory input. I firmly believe the majority of children with ASD will respond well to techniques used in a sensory processing approach. By providing you—parents, teachers, and school therapists—with descriptions of specific behavioral observations but also strategies to help provide the optimal type of input, my hope is that you'll be empowered to help your child or student become a more active participant in daily activities.

2 History and Terminology of Sensory Processing

History of Sensory Integration Therapy

The theory of sensory integration was developed by Jean Ayres, Ph.D., OTR, FAOTA, in the 1950s and has evolved over three decades (Sensory Integration and the Child, 1979). Dr. Ayres was an occupa-

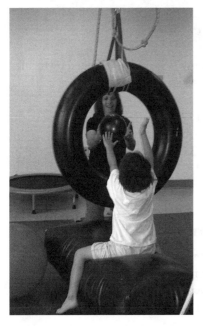

tional therapist (OT), with a doctorate in educational psychology. Following years of treating numerous individuals, she began to notice that many children shared similar abnormal behaviors in response to various types of sensory input. She began to correlate that a critical factor to a child's ongoing development was related to the integration of all the senses within the brain. "The effectiveness of a response is dependent upon the accuracy of the sensory feedback during the response" (Ayres, 1972). In simpler terms, in order for a child to begin to use his body appropriately, he must be able to take in the "just right" amount of information for the brain to determine how it needs to react. He must not only be able to use his senses in order to play with a ball, for example, but, the information must be at the "just right" level for him to be able to process in his brain and respond appropriately so he can control the ball and respond with meaning and purpose within his daily play. An inability to do this results in a lack of meaningful and purposeful interaction with one's environment.

Many occupational therapists, along with numerous other professionals (psychologists, physicians, scientists, behavioral and speech therapists, to name a few), have not only embraced Dr. Ayres's theory, they have expanded on her original findings. Extensive research continues to help validate and support the use of a sensory integrative approach to treat sensory processing disorder (SPD). Although both therapists and families have seen positive changes in their clients and children as a result of sensory integration therapy, limited research early on led many professionals, including physicians, insurance companies, and school personnel, to have doubts about whether this was a viable approach.

Ongoing research on the positive impact of using of a sensory integrative approach in children on the autistic spectrum, along with the fleshing out of Dr. Ayres's original assumptions, has continued throughout the years through the work of Lucy Jane Miller, Patricia Wilbarger, Winnie Dunn, Dr. Stanley Greenspan, and Georgia DeGangi, to name a few. Through numerous articles, ongoing research, and lectures, the terms, behaviors, and treatment of a sensory dysfunction are becoming easier to recognize and are beginning to be acknowledged by former "doubters." Current research is very exciting and many studies will help to prove and justify the use of a sensory based treatment approach as a needed and worthwhile method for helping affected children learn to function within a formerly strange world. Books detailing some of the most current research can be found in the Bibliography and Recommended Reading section at the end of this book.

Sensory Processing Terminology

Before we go on to discuss sensory dysfunction and treatment, we should first start by reviewing some of the language associated with sensory processing. So much professional jargon is bandied about in the world of sensory processing and autism and much of it can be quite confusing. What follows is a thorough discussion of the key terms that will be used throughout this book. You may choose to refer back to this chapter as a glossary while working your way through the text.

Sensory Processing

Sensory processing is a neurological process of our nervous system taking in information from our various senses (vision, hearing, touch, taste, smell, movement, and body position) **along with information from the environment** (for example, light, voices, soft toy, person standing next to you). **Information is organized in the brain, which then tells the body how to appropriately respond to the input.** Examples of normal and abnormal sensory processing systems will be illustrated and explained in depth in the next chapters.

Sensory Regulation/Modulation

The terms sensory regulation and sensory modulation are used interchangeably, and refer to **our brain's attempt to seek the "just right" level needed to attend to and organize sensory input in order to provide the best response**. Infants who are typically developing (and don't suffer from a medical condition, such as reflux) often act unsettled, crying and thrashing about, even when their basic needs have been met. This is because they haven't yet learned how to regulate their immature sensory systems. Eventually, they (and their parents) learn what works to calm them: a pacifier, bouncy seat, thumb-sucking, music, swinging, etc. Once the child is calm, he should be able to focus on his environment and begin to explore and learn.

On a daily basis, our brain is constantly trying to make sense of incoming information. To illustrate the "just right" concept, imagine a straight line running horizontally. This is considered the "just right" level of input: not too much, not too little. In other words, you're alert to changing stimuli in the background (sounds, sights, etc.) but relaxed enough to stay engaged in an activity (reading the newspaper). Until we regulate our brain to this "just right" level, it is difficult for learning to take place, as you can see from the following examples.

Imagine that our once flat line begins to go up, representing too much input, which our brain overreacts to. For example, say you're getting ready to take a very important test and the fire alarm goes off.

You are told to ignore it but you see people running for the nearest exit. Do you really think you will be able to concentrate on the test? Your focus has shifted from being calm and focused to "survival mode." A less dramatic example might be that you have had a very stressful day (sick child, toilet overflows, casserole burns). Although you manage to handle each situation, by the end of the day, you feel like your head might explode. A normal sensory system knows it needs to find ways to calm and regulate itself. For every person there are different strategies that work. Maybe you'll listen to soft classical music, dim the lights, or run a warm bath to calm your jangled nerves and bring the "line" back to horizontal.

Now picture the flat line begins to dip down. In this case, the brain is not getting enough input needed to focus on a task. Imagine, following a full work day, you have yet to prepare for a presentation you must make tomorrow. You sit at your computer unable to focus, so you get up and engage in a movement activity for five minutes and when you return, you're able to concentrate and prepare your presentation. Why did this work? Does this same strategy work for everyone? The answer is no. Just as infants learn different ways to calm or regulate their systems, so do adults. Exercise, for this person, seemed to provide the "just right" level that was needed to alert his brain and straighten the "line." Another person might use a rowing machine or vacuum the house. The main idea is that all of these types of actions provide vestibular and proprioceptive input to the brain and will improve our ability to attend and focus.

The above examples are related to a normal sensory system, whose primary job throughout the day is to determine how much is "too much" or "too little" input and adjust and regulate our nervous system to the "just right" level needed to either arouse or calm ourselves in order to attend and interact with our environment. When a child has a sensory processing disorder, he also tries to adjust the level of input, but is often unsuccessful, as we have seen with Allison in Chapter 1.

Sensory Filtering

Sensory filtering relates to our ability to determine the sensory information that is essential to complete a task and/or ignore what is not needed at that specific time. We need to be able to "filter out" all the sensory information that is bombarding our brain and concentrate only on information that is important. Children with sensory processing issues have trouble with this. They will either focus in on a very small amount of sensory information (such as having jelly on their finger, which will cause them to scream as if in severe pain until it is removed) or take in lots of information and not be able to process it (such as spinning on a toy without getting dizzy or sick). With so much sensory information bombarding us every minute of the day, our brains have quite a job of deciding how to appropriately process this information, i.e., what to pay attention to and what to ignore, depending on what we're doing.

Normal Sensory Filtering

Adam, a second grader, is taking his weekly spelling test. He sits quietly at his desk while the child next to him rustles his paper. Outside it's very windy and rain is hitting the window. Many of the children are fidgeting in their seats. However, Adam is listening for the teacher to state the next spelling word and as she does, he writes down his answer. Although there is a great deal of visual and auditory stimuli in the room, Adam's brain is filtering out unimportant information and directing his attention to listening to the teacher's voice.

Poor Sensory Filtering

Lauren, who has autism, is Adam's classmate and is also taking the spelling test. As Lauren begins to write her answer in response to the teacher, a book slips off the desk next to her. Lauren begins to fidget at her desk and hold her ears. The teacher's aide tries to calm Lauren. Lauren talks to herself, saying "It's okay, it's only a book. But I don't like the sound." The aide wraps her arm around Lauren but this only seems to upset Lauren more. She stands up and starts pacing. This is beginning to disturb the other students and the aide removes Lauren from the classroom. Once outside the room, Lauren slowly begins to calm and after a few minutes, the aide escorts Lauren back to her desk where she tries to continue to take the test. Lauren has auditory (hearing) sensitivities. She tends to over-respond to any type of auditory input, making it difficult to filter out, and preventing her from focusing on her spelling test.

Sensory Registration

Sensory registration is the ability to notice input so responses are influenced by a convergence of equally reliable sensory information

(Wilbarger & Wilbarger, 1991, revised 1997). To simplify, **sensory registration allows us to notice and interpret sensory information in a** *meaningful way* **in order to engage in the designated activity.**

Normal Sensory Registration

Gavin, a one-year-old, is seated in his high chair in front of a plate of bite-sized waffles with butter and a little syrup on top. He reaches for a piece and, upon picking it up, drops it and looks at his fingers. Confused, he licks his fingers then smears them across his tray. He then picks up a piece of waffle and brings it to his mouth. Half goes in and the rest falls on his face and chest. He likes the taste and eagerly picks up more pieces, getting some into this mouth, but mostly dropping them on himself or the floor.

After a few weeks of eating solid food, Gavin becomes much more efficient at getting his food to his mouth and the messiness has decreased considerably. His mother provides him with a small toddler spoon. Gavin tries repeatedly to scoop up waffles with his new tool. Efforts are cumbersome and success is limited; however, he continues to pursue. Usually, he will pick up the waffle pieces with his fingers and place them on the spoon. By the time he brings the spoon to his mouth, the waffle has usually fallen off and Gavin becomes somewhat frustrated. He returns to using his fingers but after a few more bites, picks up the spoon and tries again.

A few weeks later, Gavin's mother notices that he is using the spoon with more skill and less frustration. However, with any new type of food, he again tends to use his fingers if his success with the spoon isn't instant.

The above example demonstrates how a child with a normal sensory processing system learns to use a spoon. You can see that this does not happen overnight but requires a lengthy series of registering various types of sensory information (squishy waffle, sticky fingers, metal spoon, etc.). As a child continues to notice and acknowledge new input, he can begin to develop the foundation skills needed to master the total skill. Although Gavin did not initially like the sticky feeling of the syrup, he slowly began to tolerate it and kept providing his face and hands with the input. This increased tolerance enabled him to pick up the food and slowly improve his finger feeding skills. Eventually he learned to hold the spoon and control it in order to get the food to his mouth.

Registration of sensory input allows a child to focus on the activity at hand. The child is more willing to continue to try to use objects in different and more novel ways. This constant trial and error is the brain's way of learning how much movement and strength is needed to move the hand to the mouth. The final product (in this case, self-feeding with a spoon) is known as praxis, which is the ability to plan or perform a motor movement or task and is based on the ability to adequately process sensory information.

Poor Sensory Registration

Three-year-old Morgan does not like to touch or hold objects in his hands. If we place Morgan in the same scenario (eating waffles), we can imagine how he will respond. Placing his fingers on a sticky waffle will most likely send him "over the edge." When there is too much sensory input for him to comfortably process, he appears to almost shut down (turns head, hums, refuses to eat). His family will most likely try not to stress him out as they want him to gain weight and remain healthy. However, avoiding all of this sensory input will likely affect Morgan's ability to achieve higher level learning skills, such as holding objects, feeling textures, and learning how to self-feed and socialize at the dinner table.

Sensory Integration

Sensory integration is the ability of the brain to gather information from all sensory systems, along with the environment, and organize this information with the goal of *effectively planning and executing an adaptive response* to vari-ous situations. An adaptive response is the ability to respond purposefully to a situation. For example, a child who is running circles around his playroom trips over a toy. He gets up and continues to run but as he nears the toy the next time around, he adapts his response and runs around the toy. A child with poor sensory integration will most likely continue to trip over

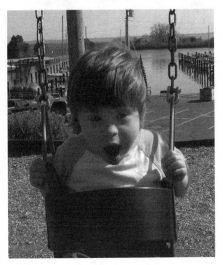

the same toy. An adaptive response is always dictated by the specific circumstances of a task. For a child with autism, an adaptive response may be tolerating sitting on a swing and holding the ropes (when previously he would not even sit on a swing). **Sensory integration** helps us learn to use our sensory systems appropriately in order to achieve optimal functioning throughout the day and **is the end result of sensory processing and sensory regulation/modulation.**

Normal Sensory Integration

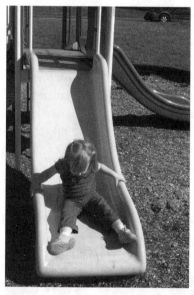

Eighteen-month-old Gavin is at the playground with his father. He has never been on a slide before. His father holds his hand and helps him climb the steps. He goes up the steps slowly, holding tightly to his father's hand. Once at the top, he seems somewhat fearful and his father supports him as he slides to the bottom. Once his feet hit the ground, he begins to laugh and asks to do it again. This time, he quickly climbs the stairs himself. At the top, he holds onto the sides of the slide and pushes off on his own. Because Gavin is able to regulate his sensory system effectively, he can process the information from the tactile input (sitting on the slide), proprioceptive input (climbing the ladder), and vestibular input (going down the slide). This process allows him to organize his behavior so he not only enjoys the sliding board experience but feels confident to increase his sliding repertoire. With each trial, Gavin demonstrates more skill and begins to try different things with the slide. Every time Gavin performs this task, his brain responds adaptively to the information from his sensory system and the environment in order for him to master the task. This is sensory integration.

Poor Sensory Integration

Morgan also enjoys going to the playground but his parents note that although he approaches the slide and swings, he rarely goes on the equipment. *He tends to push or spin the swings and will jump up and down excitedly as the swing moves. Similarly, he will run toward the slide, slap the bottom of it, and run away laughing. If his family doesn't intervene, he will continue to do this for long periods of time. When his parents attempt to place Morgan on the slide or swing, he will wriggle his body out of their grasp and run away. Morgan is unable to regulate his sensory system effectively in order to process the input from it and the environment so he can learn to use the playground equipment appropriately. He has a sensory processing dysfunction, which must be addressed before sensory integration (the end product) can take place.*

Sensory (Integration) Dysfunction

Sensory dysfunction describes the condition in which a person's brain is unable to process or organize sensory information from either the body or the environment in an appropriate or effective manner, so he's not receiving the "just right" amount of information in order to perform a specific task or behave in an appropriate manner. To paraphrase Dr. Jean Ayres: Sensory integration dysfunction is sort of like a 'traffic jam' in the brain. Some bits of sensory information get 'tied up' in traffic, and certain parts of the brain do not get the sensory information they need to do their jobs. (Ayres, 1979). In addition to not being able to perform specific tasks, a person with sensory dysfunction may engage in inappropriate behavior. For example, if a child overreacts, or is over-responsive, a little bit of information will be perceived as too much—light touch may be perceived as painful. If a child under-reacts, or is under-responsive—he craves lots of information but it does not register properly in his brain. This is most likely the child who is always touching objects or "in your face." People can exhibit over-responsive reactions, under-responsive reactions, or a combination of the two.

Sensory Processing Disorder (SPD) (Miller & Lane, 2000)

There are many different terms being used to describe this problem, such as sensory integration dysfunction and sensory modulation disorder, to name a few. For this book, the term sensory processing disorder or its acronym, SPD, will be used, as this is the terminology most widely accepted in the field. SPD is recognized as a **condition** in which a person is unable to process, regulate, and organize incoming sensory information, resulting in a poor or absent adaptive response. Generally, behavioral responses are either an over-reaction (defensive) or under-reaction (ignoring) to the sensory input. (A thorough explanation of these types of responses will be covered in Chapter 3.)

What is the difference between Sensory Integration Dysfunction (SID) and Sensory Processing Disorder/Dysfunction (SPD)?

The terms sensory integration dysfunction and sensory processing disorder (sometimes dysfunction) are often used interchangeably, but are they the same thing? The phrase sensory integration dysfunction was first coined by Dr. Jean Ayres, who was a researcher and developed the theory of Sensory Integration. The term was used to present her theory (sensory integration) but was also used to describe the type of treatment approach she developed (sensory integration therapy, or SI therapy) based on motor learning and use of an enriched environment. The idea behind sensory integration therapy is that the child is provided with the "just right" level (tolerable) of sensory input in order for him to demonstrate an adaptive response.

The term sensory processing disorder is currently being used in order to differentiate the disorder from Dr. Ayres's original theory and intervention. SPD includes three primary diagnostic groups: Type I: Sensory Modulation Disorder; Type II: Sensory Based Motor Disorder; and Type III: Sensory Discrimination Disorder (Miller et al., 2004). The three groups all have a sensory component, but people with different types will have different behavioral responses to sensory input.

Sensory Over-Responsivity (SOR)

Sensory over-responsivity, sometimes referred to as sensory defensiveness, hyperresponsivity, or hypersensitivity, **is an over-responsive reaction to nonthreatening stimuli**, such as a gentle tap on one's shoulder. The child does not view this as pleasant but overreacts with behavior such as screaming, running away, or hitting. The reason being that the stimuli sent to the brain (in this case, the tap) is viewed as threatening. The brain overreacts to the perceived danger and sends a message to the body to seek out a protective response.

Sensory over-responsivity can take other forms, for example, Lauren's reaction to the book falling off the desk next to her during the spelling test (auditory defensiveness), or Morgan's resistance to holding a spoon (tactile defensiveness). Children who are over-responsive cannot tolerate certain forms of sensory input and react as if they are something to avoid. Unfortunately, their behaviors will continue to negatively affect their ability to participate in activities and perform daily living skills.

Sensory Under-Responsivity (SUR)

Sensory under-responsivity, sometimes referred to as hyporesponsivity, or hyposensitivity, **is an under-reaction to sensory input.** Children who are under-responsive will take longer to respond to sensory input, for example, they may not respond to their name being called or may not acknowledge pain, even after a fall that results in stitches or a broken bone. This happens because the stimuli sent to the brain is not being fully registered. Children who are under-responsive are referred to as **sensory-seekers**. These sensory-seekers can't get enough input and often run around aimlessly, crash into objects and people, and touch everything in sight. They may also take excessive risks, putting themselves in danger.

Sensory Diet

Treatment for a sensory processing disorder comes in the form of a sensory diet: **a planned and scheduled activity program designed to meet a child's specific sensory needs.** The "diet of sensory information" consists of strategies that will enable a child to regulate his sensory system by either calming it down or waking it up. A trained occupational therapist (OT) will attempt various types of sensory input with a child in order to find ones that calm and simultaneously alert the child so he is ready to learn. (Sensory diet strategies are overviewed in Chapter 1 of this book and are discussed in more detail in Chapters 7, 9, and 10.)

Autism Spectrum Disorder (ASD) Terminology

Having discussed terminology associated with a sensory processing disorder, we should also review some terms often associated with autism. Since many "autistic-like" behaviors mimic those behaviors resulting from poor sensory integration, this should help you tease out what motivates your child's various behaviors so you can determine the best treatment methods.

Perseveration

Continuing to repeat a vocalization or action, such as flapping one's arms or lining up objects, **after it is no longer appropriate.** Perhaps motivated by an exaggerated need for sameness, perseverative actions will interfere with a child's ability to attend to his environment and learn.

Stereotypy or Stereotypical Behaviors (STB)

Behavior that is continually repeated with no particular purpose. Examples could be rocking, spinning objects, or repeating the same word over and over. Stereotypical behaviors are thought to be ritualistic and a rigid way to control one's environment rather than a child's attempt to modulate his sensory system. (Berkson, Guthermothe & Barabejm, 1995).

Self-Stimulation Behavior (SSB)

Persistent, repetitious abnormal behavior, thought to be a person with autism's attempt to self-modulate or arouse his sensory system, as he often has difficulty maintaining that "just right" level. (Lovaas, Newsom & Hickmanm, 1987). Self-stimulatory behaviors may look like stereotypies but are performed as a way to calm or alert the sensory system (e.g., rocking to calm, shaking hand in front of a light source to alert).

Self-injurious behaviors (SIB)

Like self-stimulation, self-injurious behaviors are **thought to be a person with autism's way of stimulating his over- or underactive sensory system in an abnormal attempt to alert or calm his sensory system.** These self-inflicted behaviors are harmful to the child and may include hair pulling, head banging, and biting.

Conclusion

Children with autism often have a sensory processing disorder. They will often display a combination of over- and under-responses (both of which will be described in great detail in the Chapter 3). Children with autism have difficulty regulating their sensory systems and, as a result, demonstrate poor sensory processing skills and sensory integration does not occur. Upon reviewing all of the sensory terminology, one can imagine how a lack of any of the components of a normal processing system will affect your child's ability to understand and process sensory information effectively. Although there is no known cure for autism, being able to identify a sensory processing disorder, along with use of various sensory strategies (deep pressure, gentle rocking, vibration, to name a few) will enable your child to begin to regulate his sensory system and process sensory information more effectively, thereby improving his daily functioning at home, school, and in the community.

The brain locates, sorts, and orders sensations—somewhat as
a traffic officer directs moving cars. When sensations flow in a
well-organized or integrated manner, the brain can use those
sensations to form perceptions, behaviors, and learning. When
the flow of sensations is disorganized, life can be like a rush hour
traffic jam.

—Jean Ayres, 1979

Sensory processing is the brain's ability to organize and make
sense of all types of sensation that enter the brain. The major portion
of the brain that is responsible for processing this input is the brainstem, which lies between the spinal cord and the higher centers of the
brain. The brainstem is the "filtering system" through which all sensory
information passes; it determines what sensory information should be
regarded and what should be ignored.

Through our senses, i.e., vision, hearing, taste, smell, touch, and
movement, the brain receives basic information, such as the color,
shape, smell, and sound of things in the environment. Every one of
our sensory organs has receptors that help to register and relay the
appropriate information to the brain. These senses are very important
in helping us learn about and use various objects within our world. We
all know basically how the eyes, ears, nose, and mouth work, but how
about touch (tactile) and the other two very important senses: vestibular (registers response to movement in relation to gravity) and proprio-

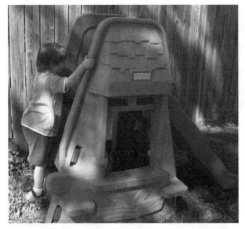

ception (registers contraction and stretching of muscles and helps us identify where our body is in relation to space)? Both the vestibular and proprioceptive senses are essential; not only for adequately processing sensory information, but for helping us learn how to control our bodies and their interactions with our environment. Their contribution consists of helping us coordinate our eyes, head, neck, and body. They also control our ability to sit erect and balance our bodies. Both of these systems are major contributors to motor planning (steps to perform a task), such as getting in and out of a car, going up and down steps, or kicking a ball.

Tactile

Just under the skin are receptors that gather information through touch. This network of receptors, known as the tactile system, is the largest sensory system. The tactile system is essential for helping us determine types of input touching our body, and how we should respond to that input (reaction as pleasant or a sensation to be avoided). Through the use of our tactile system, we are able to discriminate whether things are hot, cold, rough, smooth, etc. By touching objects, we learn to identify characteristics like size and shape and we begin to make sense of an item and its purpose. Tactile refers to all sensations through our skin.

A small child first begins to learn about his world through mouthing objects. A parent may frequently remark that "everything goes into his mouth." Mouthing objects actually helps the child understand many properties of that object through taste, texture, and size. As he grows, he begins to explore objects more through the touch of his hands versus his mouth. He may grab a rattle and hold it in his hands. He may then shake or bang the rattle, which may produce a sound or possibly give him additional information about how heavy the object may be and whether it is soft or hard.

Discriminatory touch can also be demonstrated by placing your hand in your pocket, and without use of your eyes, you should be able to locate a quarter and dime or three dimes and a nickel to make up thirty-five cents. Can you remember as a child being outside playing in the snow and when you took off your gloves, you usually had trouble picking up objects because your hands were cold? Remember the tingling, somewhat painful feeling when your hands began to "thaw" before they returned to normal? This illustrates the sensitivity of our tactile sensory system and how essential it is to our understanding of our environment through touch.

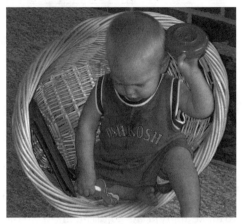

The tactile system is made up of two parts. The above description is that of discrimination—what we perceive through touching things. The majority of the receptors for discrimination are found in the fingertips but also in every other part of the body, including the tongue. The second part of our tactile system is more primitive but of utmost importance to our survival. It is the body's protective response to tactile input. It alerts the brain as to whether we should accept the input as "good" or "bad" and allows us to determine how we should react, positively or negatively ("fight or flight"). This type of touch is not usually generated by our hands but is rather how we perceive sensations around us, such as someone standing too close or touching us. An example is someone coming up behind us and grabbing our arm to get our attention. Our first reaction will likely be to withdraw and feel afraid. When we discover that it is an old friend, whom we haven't seen for a while, our sensory system will begin to relax and we re-register this touch as positive. Another type of tactile input is having your hair washed at the hairdresser. The deep pressure is most likely viewed as calming and relaxing. If you have ever had the flu or a high temperature, you can recall that feeling of your skin being "prickly" and it feels like you can feel each individual single skin cell.

Proprioception

Proprioception is our awareness of where our body is in relation to space. Information is gathered through the movement and stretching of our muscles during all types of activity, i.e., bending, pushing, pulling, etc. Imagine you are seated in a chair with your eyes closed. Now think about the position of your legs. Without looking, you can probably sense that your left ankle is crossed over your right one and your knees are touching. Proprioceptive receptors are found in the body's joints, muscles, tendons, and ligaments and are in constant communication with the brain, in order to help monitor where our body parts are without needing to look at them. This system allows us to make appropriate adjustments to balance, to move or go about daily activities without falling down or knocking into things. Have you ever imagined you were blind upon entering a dark room? Without your eyes, your entire system is "on alert" and you can sense where things are (if it is a familiar room). This is because you have a "body map" of the room from being in there numerous times with use of your vision.

Proprioception also provides deep pressure to our joints and muscles, which can be calming to the brain. We tend to seek out this type of sensory input throughout the day, most likely without thinking about it. Some examples may be tapping your leg against a chair, chewing on the tip of a pen, or enjoying the feeling of being beneath a heavy quilt for sleeping.

Vestibular

Like proprioception, this system gathers information through movement, but more in response to how our movement is affected by gravity. The vestibular system is responsible for balance and telling us the direction and speed of our body's movement. For example, if you are standing up on a crowded bus and the bus suddenly jolts, your body senses this position change. This information is processed by your vestibular system, which alerts your brain to adjust your body position

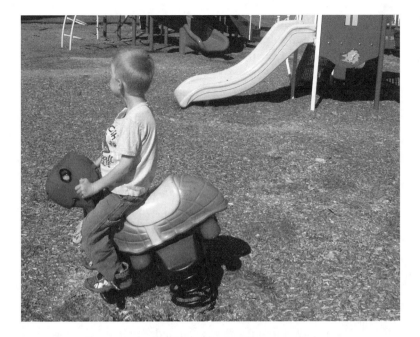

in order to keep you balanced and prevent a fall. The receptors for vestibular input are located in the inner ear, which sense movement of the head in all directions (up/down, left/right, etc). This system also works closely with the visual system in helping the brain to both see and feel where the body is in relation to objects within a room.

Do you remember as a young child standing in the center of the room and spinning and spinning until you fell down? When you stopped, the room still seemed to be spinning. Although this was a fun activity, it is not something that you'd continue to do for any lengthy period of time. This is an example of an activity that stimulates (alert) the vestibular system. Some people actually crave this type of input, where others avoid it, as it tends to make them nauseous. We also engage in activities that calm our vestibular system down, such as rocking in a rocking chair.

Normal Sensory Processing

Although each of the sensory systems are important on their own, they do not work independently but rather in conjunction with each other. All of the sensory information collected enables the brain to respond in an appropriate manner in order for us to understand and interact with our environment. Let's look again at what normal processing looks like:

Maria

Maria, a sixteen-month-old typically developing child, manages to move around her environment quite well. Her mother shows her a toy that, when activated, wiggles and plays a song. Maria squeals with delight as she watches the toy move and moves her body to the rhythm of the song. Her mouth opens and she starts to make sounds with the music. Maria's mother shows her how to start the toy by placing her hand over Maria's and activating the toy. Maria continues to be mesmerized by this toy and each time it is activated she attempts new movements, such as kicking her feet or wiggling her arms and body. By the fifth trial, she is up and spinning around and falling when she becomes dizzy. She laughs. Her arms reach out to catch herself as she falls. With each trial, she continues to add new actions. Maria's overall skills, such as balance and movement, become more and more refined the longer she interacts with this object.

To further illustrate the orchestration of all the senses, let's look more carefully at Maria's entire sensory processing system as she interacts with the musical toy. Maria is drawn to and curious about the colorful toy (**vision**). She enjoys the music emitted from the toy (**auditory**). She is provided deep pressure (mother's hand on top of hers) in order to understand how to activate the toy (both **tactile** and **proprioceptive**). She does not passively watch the toy's actions, but actively responds physically with her body. She tries to imitate the actions of the toy by kicking her feet and wiggling her body (**proprio-ception**). Trying to spin and turn her body (**vestibular**), she is not only experiencing the movement, but with each trial, the information that is being sent to her brain is being returned with data that is helping her refine her movements.

The above information is mostly being viewed from a physical point of view. However, the major component that permits Maria to engage in this task is that she feels comfortable with information from her tactile system and perceives this as a "safe" place and activity. Her mother's touch is viewed as one of comfort and pleasure. Her brain is registering this information and relating that there is no danger and she can be comfortable (**modulation**) and focus on the actions of the toy. Maria is able to attend to the sensory information pertaining to the toy rather than all other input from around the room (TV on, dog barking, etc.). This is an example of the brain's ability to **filter** out unimportant information and focus only on information related to the task.

Abnormal Sensory Processing

Although children with autism are not the only ones who struggle with SPD, they do seem to be affected in a disproportionably high number. Children with autism have all the sensory systems listed above. If a physician could test their sensory systems, likely, the results would indicate everything was working just fine. But, are they? If so, why do they often avoid eye contact or stare into lights? Why do they sometimes act as though they are deaf or the opposite: begin to scream and hold their ears at everyday sounds? Why do some refuse to hold toys in their hands and seem happiest to sit and spin the toy for long periods of time? How come some can spin and spin and never appear dizzy? Why do they only eat certain foods? In the following section, we will examine how children with autism may perceive or interpret sensory information, which might provide some explanation for some of their "odd" behaviors.

Evan

Evan is an eight-year-old boy who was diagnosed with classic autism at the age of three. Evan uses only a limited vocabulary to communicate, hates to have his routine changed, is a picky eater (only eats certain foods at certain times), will only wear certain types of clothing, and becomes easily upset (screams, runs away) for what appears to be no reason. He does not play with toys and engages in many self-stimulatory behaviors. (Self-stimulation describes when a child performs a certain movement with no real purpose over and over again.) For example, Evan will shake his fingers back and forth in front of a light source. He also does this with Mardi Gras beads. When Evan is doing this activity, he will laugh and rock to the action. This appears "fun" for Evan and he becomes upset if someone takes the beads away or tries to hold his hands down. He also becomes very upset if someone tries to either talk or play with him during these times.

Although Evan demonstrated many of these behaviors as a young child, his family has recently become more concerned with his decreased participation in daily activities (dressing, self-feeding) along with his refusal to play with toys or hold a pencil. He is also showing an increase in self-injurious behaviors, including banging his head, screaming, and hitting and biting himself. School is reporting increased frustration with his behaviors and Evan's family is fearful that as he becomes older, they will be unable to handle him.

Evan is about to participate in his first occupational therapy (OT) appointment. His family arrives five minutes early and they are asked to wait in the waiting room. The room is a long hallway with other families also waiting for their appointments. Evan's mother leads Evan to a chair and as she holds his hand, she feels his body tense. He sits and starts to rock in a rhythmic pattern, but after about a minute, he starts to rock harder and make loud humming noises. As she tries to quiet him, Evan's voice becomes louder and he starts to run up and down the hallway. His behavior becomes so out of control, that he is escorted into a small treatment room. By this time, he is unable to be calmed and the OT questions his mother about what may help. She explains that he likes to watch Barney videos while jumping on a trampoline. Fortunately, both a video and a trampoline are available and after about three minutes, Evan begins to calm and they are able to begin the session.

Although Evan has all the same sensory systems as Maria, from our earlier case study, Evan's are not functioning appropriately, and as a result, he is unable to make sense of sensory information. As various types of information (other children sitting in chairs waiting for their appointments, parents talking, fluorescent lighting, the smell of new carpet, etc.) enter Evan's brain, he is unable to determine a correct response and as a result, his behavioral responses are inappropriate and puzzling to the average person.

Are all of Evan's behaviors related to his having autism or are some behaviors related to a sensory processing disorder? Many children who have a sensory processing disorder without autism may exhibit odd behaviors, such as the examples given above. A possible explanation is that even though a child is unable to process sensory information effectively, the brain still demands a response to sensory information. Many children, like Evan, will seek out sensory input, such as moving a hand in front of a light source. This may seem "weird" to us, but it is actually Evan's attempt to provide "seeing" and "touching" information to his brain. Although abnormal, it is his way of trying to make sense" of the world. Unfortunately, it is not functional and because he is obsessed with this stimulus, he will often refuse to participate in any "normal" type of activities. You can see how this will affect his everyday life.

Evan's family and school were hoping that as he grew older, these rituals would decrease; however, just the opposite has happened: they have become part of his daily routine. Although Evan's primary diagnosis is autism, many of his behaviors appear to be sensory-based. This chapter will explain various components of an abnormal sensory system.

Why Does Sensory Dysfunction Happen?

Our brains are constantly being bombarded with information from all of the senses. Not only must the brain try to decipher data, but it must respond to input in an agreeable or "just right for the situation" manner, in order to produce an adaptive response. For example, you are sitting in a room and a strange sound comes from outside the door. Your adaptive response is to turn your eyes and head towards the sound. For this to happen, the brain seeks a "just right" level (modulation) necessary for you to attend to and organize the sensory input. In this case, the "just right" level means you remain calm and use your vision and hearing to help determine the cause of the sound and how you should respond.

For children with a sensory processing disorder (SPD), information coming into the brain is either perceived as "too much" or "not enough." **An over-responsive system perceives incoming information to the brain as "too much"; an under-responsive system sees it as "too little."** The result for either extreme is an inappropriate response to stimuli. In the literature, different terms may be used for these conditions. Over-responsive may be referred to as "hyperresponsive," "hypersensitive," or "over-aroused," and under-responsive may be called "hyporesponsive," "hyposensitive," or "under-aroused." In this book, the terms over-responsive and under-responsive will primarily be used.

It should be noted that a child can have a combination of some over- and under-responsive behaviors. This is very common in children with autism and creates confusion when trying to determine the cause of many of their abnormal responses to situations. For example, your child may become very upset by the sound of a clock ticking in the next room, but not respond to you calling his name loudly. How a child responds to the same stimuli from one day to the next may also fluctuate.

Over-Responsive Reaction to Sensory Stimuli

An over-responsive system will react to very small amounts of information entering the brain and will perceive it as a reason to react negatively or avoid it. Someone with a "normal" sensory processing system may initially be very aware of any new type of input, such as someone nearby talking loudly on a cell phone, but eventually "tune out" or ignore the input and focus on more important things. Children with an over-responsive system overreact to everyday input and never seem to feel comfortable with various sensations. This over-responsive state may illicit a behavioral reaction from one specific sense, like hearing, or it may spill over to numerous senses, such as vision, movement, etc.

In the case study above, Evan is expected to sit patiently in a crowded waiting room. The sounds that he hears, the children in the room, and the unfamiliar environment are all perceived by him as threatening. Evan is demonstrating an over-responsive reaction to various types of stimuli in the waiting room, including auditory, tactile, and olfactory. He has difficulty processing just one sound, let alone many types of sounds and people around him talking simultaneously. The noises, the proximity of people sitting next to him, the scratchy feel of the fabric on the chair, smells from clothing, deodorant, etc., all prove to be too much for his sensory systems to handle. When a child's mind is in an over-responsive state, he is unable to focus on anything other than those particular stimuli. Evan's brain is unable to decipher the information in an appropriate manner and, as a result, his brain assumes a defensive mode. His sympathetic nervous system is in overdrive. Exhibiting a protective response may cause his behavior to escalate to the point of being out of control. He is likely to demonstrate either a "fight" (hitting or pushing) or "flight" (running around the room) reaction. If a child is always in a state of "fight or flight," he will likely suffer from anxiety and chronic stress, and it will be very difficult for him to engage in everyday activities, such as eating, dressing, holding objects, and interacting with people.

Common Over-Responsive Behaviors

Tactile Defensiveness

Tactile defensiveness is an over-reaction to touch. Very small amounts of tactile input, like a gentle tap on the shoulder or the feeling of someone's body brushing against yours, are "over-registered" by the over-responsive brain, perceived as painful or dangerous, and produce a heightened reaction. This perception affects a child's ability to perform daily living skills and participate in activities at home, school, and in the community. The brain is registering the tactile defensive response and is always "on alert" rather than getting used to these everyday types of sensory input.

Tactile defensiveness can also affect a child's use of his hands to hold objects. Due to the brain's over-response, the child will avoid touching objects and, as a result, not receive the important information needed to play with or use objects (necessary to learn). This can also affect his interactions with family members and in social situations, in that, if another child is either standing too close or approaches him to play, he will overreact and possibly strike out or run away to avoid contact (fight or flight response).

Common Manifestations of Tactile Defensiveness.
- May only wear long-sleeved shirts and long pants throughout the year
- Wears only very old, worn-out clothing with soft seams
- May prefer minimal amount of clothing; tend to strip down
- May prefer snug-fitting clothing, e.g., leotards, leggings, etc.
- Pulls tags out of clothes
- Hates having body washed, especially hair, face, and teeth brushed
- Appears hyperactive (running around), usually in an attempt to avoid or escape tactile input
- Avoids playing with other children in class or playground
- Needs a lot of personal space; may hit or push a person standing too close to him

- Difficulty with group activities like "circle time"
- Hates having hair cut
- Avoids any manipulation activities with his hands
- Hates to be messy
- Avoids writing and drawing tasks
- Avoids messy play like painting or gluing

Oral Defensiveness

Oral defensiveness can also be classified under tactile defensiveness as food avoidance, and may be related to over-registration of tactile input to the mouth. Although we all have food preferences, a child with oral defensiveness has extreme responses to food. Many times, a child will avoid food with any texture and may eat only soft foods, such as yogurt or pudding. He could have a significant amount of difficulty graduating to more complex and age-appropriate foods (such as sandwiches, hamburgers, vegetables) as he ages. Often, even the smallest amount of two combined textures (e.g., cracker crumbs mixed into pudding) may cause gagging or vomiting. Due to the over-sensitivities associated with oral input, a child might react with avoidance, screaming, or refusal to eat. These children are often extremely vigilant about their food and become upset if offered any new type of food.

Therapy designed to help a child overcome his oral defensiveness is usually a very slow, gradual process. Often a preferred taste (for example ketchup or chocolate) is identified and used by the therapist to entice the child to begin to tolerate minute pieces of texture (mixed in with the preferred taste) and gradually "working up" to more complex ones. You can see how this type of behavior will also affect the social aspects of a meal, which we usually perceive as a pleasant experience. (Food selectivity and oral defensiveness are discussed in more detail in Chapters 5 and 9.)

Common Manifestations of Oral Defensiveness.
- Hates having teeth brushed, face washed
- Gags on any type of texture or "chunk" in food
- Becomes upset if food is on his face
- May be a picky eater; prefers to stick to same types of food
- Tends to eat mostly bland food
- Keeps foods separated on his plate (doesn't want them to touch)

Olfactory Defensiveness

Imagine you are on a crowded elevator with someone who has strong body odor. Likely, you will be greatly focused on this until you are able to get off the elevator and breathe some fresh air. This is equivalent to what some children, who have an over-responsive sense of smell, deal with all the time. In a room full of people, the smell of perfume, deodorant, gasoline on someone's hands, and so on, bombard their sensory systems. If a child is over-responsive to smell, this has the potential to affect his ability to focus on schoolwork and activities, as well as socializing and enjoying an event.

We know that smell and taste go hand in hand. Not surprisingly, a child's olfactory defensiveness can greatly affect his eating habits and food preferences. I once knew a young boy with autism who went to stay with his aunt for a week. By the middle of the week, his aunt called the boy's parents and reported that her nephew would only eat finger foods and refused to use utensils. When asked why he would not use his aunt's silverware, he said it had a "funny smell." The solution was to use plastic silverware since his nose did not register it as noxious as the regular silverware.

Common Manifestations of Olfactory Defensiveness.

- Often upset, agitated, or distracted by certain scents, especially strong, chemical scents, such as cleaning products or new clothing smells
- May refuse to use utensils if not familiar to him
- Gags or vomits on certain odors, food tastes, or toothpaste
- May become nauseous or develop headaches from certain smells

Auditory Defensiveness

Auditory defensiveness is an over-reaction to noise. Although we may initially react to a novel, strange, or especially loud sound (e.g., work crew outside drilling the street, sudden noise from a door slamming, low battery alert from a fire detector), children who are hypersensitive to sound have difficulty with some everyday sounds, even relatively quiet ones. This is seen in the above description of Evan in the waiting room at the OT's office. The noises, among other things, are not perceived as pleasant but rather very disturbing or even painful. His response is to race back and forth and hum loudly, possibly to drown out the other noises. A hyperreaction to sound can affect simple family gatherings, such as going out to "fun" places, like McDonald's, the mall, family celebrations, and other places that are typically crowded and noisy.

Common Manifestations of Auditory Defensiveness.
- Can become upset with "everyday" noises, such as children talking, vacuum cleaner, clock ticking, toilet flushing, dog barking
- Visibly upset by loud but familiar sounds (school bell, toilet flushing, fire engine)
- May become upset if the radio is not "tuned in"
- Cannot handle crowds and large group activities
- May actually turn up the radio or TV very loud in an effort to block out other sounds
- Becomes very anxious and alert to the anticipation of sounds from school PA systems, toilets flushing, etc.

Visual Defensiveness

Visual defensiveness is an over-reaction to visual information. In this case, the brain is unable to process the abundance of visual information in a busy environment. Some children may cry or over-react to increased visual stimuli or retreat to a darkened area. Others may respond by staring intently at an object in an abnormal attempt to block out visual stimuli. This will negatively affect a child's eye-hand coordination needed to play, eat, and participate in school activities.

Some children with autism may also suffer from Irlen syndrome, characterized by a visual perceptual problem caused by hypersensitivity to color, lights, glare, patterns, and contrast. Although there is some controversy surrounding its diagnostic criteria and treatment methods, the Irlen Institute estimates that this syndrome may affect up to half of the autistic population (Irlen, 1991).

Common Manifestations of Visual Defensiveness.
- Avoids eye contact (possibly due to too much visual stimuli on people's faces)
- Often uses peripheral vision (looks at things out of the corners of the eyes)
- Closes eyes in response to light glare, colors, etc.

- Gets upset by bright lights (fluorescent)
- Easily distracted by visual stimuli (e.g., flickering fluorescent light)
- May prefer to be in darkened areas
- May get distracted or irritated by clutter (including busy patterns and too many bright colors)
- Tends to like things kept the same way (e.g., furniture placement)

Gravitational Insecurity

The vestibular system is responsible for processing movement in response to the pull of gravity. It tells us when to use a protective response (be careful!) and when it's okay to engage in a movement. It lets us know where our body is in relation to space. A child who experiences gravitational insecurity perceives movement as "scary" and usually responds to it with exaggerated emotionality. Our sense of gravity will usually alert us when we are going to fall but for a child with this type of hypersensitivity, the response is way out of proportion. These kids tend to be observers and do not readily engage in activities that require movement. They prefer to be close to the ground and usually will not venture off to try anything new. They are able to manage a task, such as sitting on a swing with their feet on the ground, but once their feet come off the ground, they're not able to understand where their bodies are in relation to space. Even though they are inches above the ground, their perception may be that of falling off the edge of a cliff. This is usually a child who becomes upset at playgrounds, on carnival rides, or going up or down open steps.

Common Manifestations of Gravitational Insecurity.
- Avoids activities that involve movement, especially those in which the feet are not on stable ground (e.g., swinging, riding a bike)
- Does not like going up or down steps or escalators
- Prefers to be close to the ground (lying down, seated)
- Avoids playground activities with fast movements, such as tag or playing ball
- Does not like carnival rides
- May experience motion sickness (especially on car rides)
- Seems to move stiffly or holds body in awkward or fixed movement patterns

- Often does not like the daily routine or environment changed

Abnormal Compensations of an Over-Responsive Sensory System

Although the brain of a child with an over-responsive system overreacts to input, it is still trying (in its abnormal way) to make sense of sensory input and enable the body to respond appropriately. A child with autism and SPD will usually exhibit "strange" compensatory behaviors in an effort to help him calm down. Many of the behaviors become habits that continue even after the original distress has passed. In the example of Evan, his way to self-calm was to hum and rock and to distract himself with a specific video and jump on a trampoline.

As we have said, a child who has an over-sensitive response is in protective mode. The brain is on high alert and unable to make sense of the incoming stimuli and the child tends to react by crying, screaming, hitting, avoiding, or running away. We often see the child attempting to calm or regulate his system by engaging in behaviors that may appear senseless. Although "inappropriate" reactions, these behaviors are familiar to us as expressions of the "fight or flight" mode—a primal response wherein we either stay and fight or run away.

Below are lists of some behaviors seen in children with hypersensitivities and a possible explanation for what type of input they may be craving. Although some of these behaviors result from a child's autism, we want to begin to "tease out" whether sometimes these behaviors are symptomatic of SPD and are the child's attempt to help regulate his sensory system. Children with over-responsive systems will likely seek out deep pressure or auditory feedback as a means to calm themselves.

Deep pressure and proprioceptive input, depending upon the way it is used, can be calming to the brain and this type of input may help an over-responsive child settle down. Examples of children seeking this type of input can take the form of:
- Pacing back and forth
- Pushing against a wall or other stationary object
- Knocking over heavy objects
- Jumping up and down
- Rocking back and forth

- Flapping arms and clapping hands
- Needing to always hold onto a specific toy (stuffed animal, plastic toy) and rub it in a specific manner

Auditory feedback is also reported to be calming to the brain. Examples of children seeking this type of input can take the form of:
- Humming
- Grinding teeth
- Making strange and repetitive sounds
- Chewing on plastic or non-edible objects, especially clothing (even if they have oral defensiveness)
- Scripted language (e.g., from TV shows, commercials)

The following are often done as a means to decrease the amount of *visual or auditory input* in order to calm oneself:
- Retreating to a darkened corner
- Finding a quiet and vacant part of the house (closet, behind the sofa, laundry basket)
- Rolling up inside a large, heavy quilt or blanket
- Avoiding social or eye contact
- Staring into a light source in order to block out other visual stimuli
- Putting hands over ears or screaming in an effort to block out other auditory stimuli

Throughout the day and over our lifetime, we all experience various types of input that can cause us to overreact, for example, roller coasters, slimy foods, messy hands, etc. This does not mean we all have a sensory processing issue. Although we may register certain input as uncomfortable, our sensory systems are functioning normally, and we are still able to go about our day and function within a normal manner. Likewise, some of the behaviors that we've classified as "abnormal compensations" can also be seen in typically developing children and are developmentally normal. Unfortunately, for children who are sensory defensive, their reaction to everyday stimuli is perceived as painful or dangerous and will, most likely, affect their daily activities at home, school, and in the community. Because they avoid a world full of sensory experiences, they are prevented from interacting with people and objects as one would expect.

"There is a part of the brain that is concerned with the desire to initiate behavior, to respond to sensory stimuli, to do something new or different. This part of the brain has an energizing effect; it says, 'Do it!' to the parts of the brain that tell the muscles to move the body....Like the system that registers sensations, the "I want to do it" system is working poorly in the autistic child. (Ayres, 1979)

Under-Responsive Reaction to Sensory Stimuli

In the case of a child with an under-responsive system, large amounts of information enter the brain but are not processed, so the brain keeps sending out the message to "give it more information." This sensation-seeking inclination might manifest itself as hyperactivity and impulsivity.

A young, typically developing child will pick up a new toy and touch and look at it. After a few seconds, he will usually try to do something with the toy (i.e., push it, roll it) until he gets a reaction or satisfaction from the object. A child who is tactilely under-responsive may appear to do the same as this other child but his attempts to play with the toy are usually haphazard. The child with the under-responsive system never appears to gather enough sensory information to produce an adaptive response necessary to play with or use the toy in an appropriate manner. His response may be to either throw the object or otherwise avoid the task. A child experiencing an under-responsive reaction may be described as a "clumsy child" who is often tripping over the same item or bumping into people or objects.

Jasmine

Jasmine is in a preschool gymnastics program. Although it seems she enjoys the class, she isn't able to participate in a typical way. She has trouble using the gym equipment and often resorts to rolling on the floor. Or, instead of joining her classmates and playing on the equipment, she'll run circles around the room. She does not follow the instructor's directions and instead crashes into things and throws herself on the gym mats, often disrupting the other children. She's always touching people or objects. If she picks up a ball, she throws it with a great deal of force, seemingly unaware that she could hurt someone. Many times, she will push a child who is in her way and not respond to the child's reaction. She often becomes very silly and laughs nervously.

When efforts are made to calm her, Jasmine becomes sillier and appears unable to follow directions. The instructor cannot continue the class as all energy is focused on getting Jasmine to settle down and behave. As a result, she is placed in a quiet "time out" area and, after a few minutes, is able to return to the group. However, once back with the group, the same behaviors occur again and her mother is often called in to remove Jasmine. This continues to concern Jasmine's mother. If she can't even handle a small gym class, what will life be like when it's time for Jasmine to attend school?

Many of Jasmine's behaviors are abnormal responses to every-day activities. Because Jasmine communicates verbally very well and appears to be able to understand what she is being told, it's easy to assume she's misbehaving on purpose. This is not the case. Her brain is simply not interpreting specific sensory information in a meaningful way. Jasmine gets "set off" when she experiences activities that involve movement. It seems that the more sensory input she receives, particularly vestibular, proprioceptive, and tactile, the more she craves.

Jasmine is a sensory-seeker. She is constantly moving and seeking out input from movement and touch, but is unable to register it adequately and, unfortunately, her behaviors are not conducive to being able to interact with her peers. Interestingly, sometimes children who have under-responsive sensory systems might withdraw and appear lethargic—they do not notice or respond to sensation. In both of these cases, the brain is not able to filter and register the "just right" amount of input in order to come up with an adaptive response. This explains why, for example, some under-responsive kids will crave spicy food while others tend to eat mostly bland food.

Common Under-Responsive Behaviors

Tactile Under-Responsiveness

The tactically under-responsive child can be driven to constantly touch objects, yet has difficulty processing information through holding or manipulating objects. Large amounts of sensory input (proprioceptive, tactile, etc.) enter the brain, but the child is unable to register or process it correctly and as a result does not get the "right" feedback to use a crayon or spoon, for example. A child with tactile under-responsivity will hold objects, but his grasp may be awkward or clumsy. Children who are under-responsive may not respond to pain or extreme temperatures and are at risk of harming themselves.

Common Manifestations of Tactile Under-Responsivity.
- Messy eating habits
- Unaware of food on face or messy hands
- Clothing is often disheveled
- Difficulty with managing fasteners
- Difficulty using small tools like spoons, crayons, scissors (grip can be too strong or too weak)
- Seems to be always touching objects
- May be unaware of extreme pain or temperature changes

Oral Under-Responsivity
A child who is orally under-responsive will constantly put things in his mouth, such as toys, fingers, or food. Although all the oral motor aspects (chew, swallow) are intact, the child may not be registering the sensations and, in an effort to get more input, may display odd behaviors, such as chewing on clothes, blankets, and such.

Common Manifestations of Oral Under-Responsivity.
- Stuffs food in mouth; unaware of too much food in mouth
- Prefers bland foods
- Drools past the expected age
- Chews food too much or too little
- Has difficulty drinking from a cup
- Craves spicy or strong flavored food
- Puts unusual or non-edible items in mouth

Olfactory Under-Responsivity
A child with an under-responsive system may be driven to taste or smell everything. He also may not acknowledge strong smells like chemicals or smoke. Again, although massive amounts of sensory information are entering the brain, it is not processed in a way that provides adequate information about the item.

Common Manifestations of Olfactory Under-Responsivity.
- Tastes and smells all objects before playing with them
- Tastes and smells food before eating it (beyond what is considered "normal")
- May sniff people, clothing, objects
- May seek out odd or noxious scents, e.g., cleaning products
- May ignore unpleasant odors, such as dirty diapers

Auditory Under-Responsivity

A child with an under-responsive system typically has functional hearing but his brain fails to register or respond to everyday auditory input. While all children have moments when they ignore certain noises or someone calling their name, children with an under-responsive system will do this far more often than normal. Often, parents of a child with auditory issues will be concerned about their child's hearing and even go so far as to get his hearing checked. More often than not, the sensory systems involved with hearing are just fine—it is what happens in the child's brain that is responsible for the dysfunction.

Common Manifestations of Auditory Under-Responsivity.
- May not respond to his name being called
- Ignores others' voices
- May have trouble following directions
- May talk too loud or too soft (difficulty modulating voice)
- May obsess over sounds, such as flushing the toilet
- May like TV or music louder than normal
- May make a lot of noise
- Easily distracted by noises in the room (e.g., other people talking)

Visual Under-Responsivity

The function of our visual system is not only to look at people and objects, but use our peripheral vision to know what is next to us as we move through space. A child with an under-responsive system seems to be unaware of people and things within his environment. This may possibly be related to the diagnosis of autism, as this child may use his peripheral vision more than his central. Often he'll have difficulty locating objects, especially in a visually "busy" area, and may have trouble putting on clothes (i.e., finding the arm hole on his shirt.)

Common Manifestations of Visual Under-Responsivity.
- Difficulty putting toothpaste on a toothbrush and other such tasks
- Can't find a particular item when it is "hidden" in a group of other items
- Stares at bright lights or the sun and does not register discomfort
- Attends for long periods of time to one specific visual task (flashing objects, stripes on a toy, spinning objects, etc.)
- Appears to enjoy visually stimulating environments
- May enjoy watching objects spin
- May rewind a video to a certain part over and over

Proprioceptive Under-Responsivity

Proprioception is information from our joints, muscles, tendons, and ligaments that tells us where our body is in relation to space. When a child is under-responsive to proprioceptive input, again, all the information that enters his brain is not filtered or processed correctly. He may be clumsy, always tripping over objects, or bumping into walls, mainly because he doesn't have a "body map" (knowing where his limbs and such are in relation to the environment). Often, a child with this type of under-responsivity will try to get adequate sensory information about his body by crashing and bumping into the walls or furniture in his surroundings, as seen in the case of Jasmine.

A child with a normal proprioceptive system can learn a skill step by step, for example, how to get on a swing, hold onto the ropes, and eventually pump. Over and over, this child takes the information in, processes it in his brain, and produces an adaptive response that enables him to swing. If you watch a child with a poorly functioning proprioceptive system, he will attempt the same task but be unable to produce ongoing appropriate adaptive responses, which, in turn, will affect his success with that activity.

Common Manifestations of Proprioceptive Under-Responsivity.
- Seems to always be hanging on people, leaning on walls, etc.
- Often bangs into walls and objects, seeking feedback about where he is in space

- Seems to tire before other children
- Experiences difficulty with tasks that involve dexterity, such as pouring milk
- Trips over the same items repeatedly; doesn't seem to be aware of things in his way (clumsy)
- Has difficulty learning how to dress himself and use fasteners (snaps, buttons, zippers)
- Has poor motor planning skills (ability to figure out how to get on a swing, sliding board, ride a bike, activate a toy, etc.)
- Seems to use too much force when throwing a ball, coloring with a crayon; may be considered "rough" when playing games at recess or gym class
- Craves jumping, crashing, pushing, or bouncing activities
- Doesn't provide others with appropriate personal space (stands or sits too close)
- Withdrawn, doesn't care to engage in play with peers
- Will often need to look at feet while walking, dancing, etc. (relies on vision)

Vestibular Under-Responsivity

The vestibular system is responsible for registering where our body is in relation to the pull of gravity. A child with an under-responsive vestibular system may crave movement, such as spinning his body around and around for lengthy periods of time, never complaining of dizziness or nausea. A child with a normal vestibular system will enjoy this activity for a brief period of time but will quickly become dizzy and most likely vomit if he continues. The sensory system of a child who is under-responsive craves the spinning but his brain does not know when to "shut it off" and as a result, this child does not get dizzy. He is also not registering vestibular input correctly and this will affect how his body responds to it, perhaps resulting in poor posture or weak upper arms.

Common Manifestations of Vestibular Under-Responsivity.

- Loses balance and may fall if he bends in any direction off his base of support
- Moves head in a repetitive movement
- Seeks out excessive body spinning activities; may like to spin objects too

- May become overly excited during play activities
- In an academic setting: slumps on desk or leans on arm, tires easily, has difficulty with visual tracking and loses place on the paper

Abnormal Compensations of an Under-Responsive Sensory System

As we stated in the above section, the brain continuously tries to "make sense" of the sensory information it receives. Under-responses will obviously look different than over-responses given that the brain of a child who is under-responsive allows large amounts of information to enter but is unable to discern what to pay attention to and what to ignore. As a result, the child does not get the right type of input and is unable to provide an appropriate adaptive response. A child with autism will seek out the sensory input and, again, may exhibit an abnormal or odd response. Some of the responses may be related to autism, but often, the behaviors are the child's weak attempts at trying to provide his sensory system with (what he believes) is the "just right" amount and kind of input.

Below are lists of some behaviors exhibited by children with under-responsive systems. You may notice that many of the behaviors listed are also listed in the section of common behaviors of children who are over-responsive. It's true that these children often do the same things, the difference being why: the over-responsive child is looking to calm his system, while the under-responsive child is trying to alert his system.

Proprioceptive input is reported to be alerting to the brain. Examples of children seeking this type of input can take the form of:
- Crashing into furniture and bumping into walls
- Pushing objects
- Knocking over heavy objects
- Jumping up/down
- Fast motion activities, such as swinging, jumping off high surfaces
- Flapping arms and clapping hands
- May seem lethargic or withdrawn

Depending on how it's used, *tactile input* is reported to "wake up" the brain. Examples of children seeking this type of input can take the form of:

- Chewing on clothing or nonedible objects
- Picking at a sore or biting hands
- Stuffing mouth with food
- Hitting head or body hard against a wall or surface
- Ignoring requests to wear gloves in the winter because he doesn't notice hand being cold
- Liking drastic temperature changes, such as a very hot room in the summer and the window open in the winter.

Some children with under-repsonsive sensory systems seek out *auditory input* in the form of:

- Liking very loud music and TV
- Talking very loud or making strange loud noises

Examples of children seeking *visual input* can take the form of:

- Staring at bright lights for long periods of time
- Dangling beads in front of eyes
- Spinning objects for lengthy periods of time
- Using peripheral vision
- Perseverating on a certain action of a toy
- Playing the same scene of a movie repeatedly

As with the children who are over-responsive and avoid sensory input, one can see how children who are under-responsive will have difficulty with daily activities and play. Children with autism and/or SPD seek out their version of the "just right" amount and type of sensory input, but unfortunately their attempts are usually inadequate. Because their attempts provide their brains some sort of stimuli, it is often difficult to extinguish these behaviors and allow more normal and appropriate learning to happen. For example, a child may initially look at a bright light to satisfy his under-responsive system's need for visual feedback but may soon realize that this, along with flicking his fingers in front of the light source, is pleasing to him. Getting him to look at a book or hold a spoon to self-feed will become increasingly difficult, as he will not want to stop this pleasurable visual activity. The goal of a sensory diet is to provide the child with more appropriate types of sensory stimuli (to satisfy his sensory system) so he will begin to use eyes and hands more effectively in play and daily tasks.

Conclusion

Children on the autism spectrum are not the only ones who experience SPD. There are many children with and without learning disabilities and those with AD/HD (attention deficit/hyperactivity disorder) who also demonstrate many of the behaviors described in this chapter. SPD also affects their ability to perform daily living skills, such as dressing, using a pencil, participating in sports, and interacting with their peers. The child with AD/HD and SPD will more than likely demonstrate other types of behaviors, such as having trouble finishing tasks, losing or misplacing toys, or always being "on the go." Children with AD/HD and SPD are more at risk for emotional and behavioral problems (if SPD is not addressed) because they are more aware that they "can't" participate along with their peers, so they may tend to withdraw or "act out" (hitting, talking back, refusing to participate, etc).

Children with Asperger's disorder usually have fairly good language skills and are often mainstreamed into regular classes with the help of a good support team at school. Children with Asperger's disorder can usually provide some insight into their perception of sensory processing deficits. Temple Grandin, a well-known author and a person with Asperger's disorder, has written numerous books and shared many stories about how she perceives the world, including the effect sensory processing disorder has on her life. Children with autism are usually not as aware of how their peers perceive them. The majority of these kids do not have the social and language skills to be able to convey how they feel. As a result, they will exhibit more odd-type behaviors, but hopefully, we will be able to tease out which are over- or under-responses and develop a sensory diet that allows that child to calm or alert his sensory system. Helping children learn more appropriate strategies to process sensory information should enable them to increase their participation in tasks that they have avoided. Note, however, that while many sensory strategies can help modulate a child's sensory system, this does not "cure" him of autism.

4 Does My Child Have a Sensory Processing Disorder?
The Evaluation Process

Children with an autistic spectrum disorder (ASD) demonstrate stereotypical behaviors and decreased social interaction and communication skills. Research is beginning to document that an

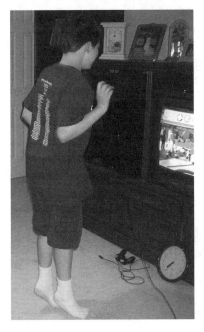 atypical sensory processing system is also a central aspect of an autistic spectrum disorder (Zoe Mailloux, 2001). Parents of children with autism often report that their child is a picky eater; hates having his face washed and teeth brushed; has difficulty with changes in seasonal clothing (i.e., wants to wear shorts in winter and long-sleeved shirts in summer); screams or acts out in new environments; refuses to hold objects in his hands; won't play with toys in a typical fashion; and likes sameness and routine. While these can be typical characteristics of a child with autism, many of these behaviors are also associated with a sensory processing disorder and it is important to have your child evaluated to determine if this is the case. If your child is diagnosed

with SPD, services can be provided to pinpoint the reasons behind the behaviors and action can be taken to treat the root cases. (See Chapter 5 for discussion of how sensory dysfunction affects your child's ability to attend, learn, play, socialize, sleep, eat, and so on.)

Look-alike Disorders

Children with autism sometimes demonstrate behaviors that are associated with other types of developmental disorders, such as Oppositional Defiant Behavior (ODD), Obsessive-Compulsive Disorder (OCD), Generalized Anxiety disorder, Traumatic Brain Injury (TBI), and Cerebral Palsy (CP).

It's easy to see where many of the characteristic behaviors of ASD, SPD, and these developmental disorders overlap. For example, if your child is over-responsive to tactile input and is asked to hold a spoon that he perceives as aversive, your child will more than likely become defiant and refuse to participate. This behavior could be perceived as typical of ODD. If your child is over-responsive to auditory input and is at the circus, he will more than likely become very anxious and overwhelmed by the situation and begin to scream or refuse to participate. This behavior could be perceived as typical of an anxiety disorder. Many children with ASD (especially those with Asperger's disorder) become obsessed with a certain subject (e.g., astronomy) and feel compelled to carry around articles associated with the subject at all times. This behavior could be perceived as typical of OCD.

It is tricky to tease out which behavioral characteristics are associated with what disorder, so it is very important to have your child evaluated by an occupational therapist (OT) who is trained in identifying a sensory processing disorder. The remainder of this chapter will break down the steps of the evaluation process and provide answers to common questions. We will discuss what the evaluation process should look like and guide you to find the most appropriate professional to conduct the evaluation and provide education and training to your family about therapeutic approaches to use with your child with SPD.

Breaking Down the Evaluation Process

Before the Evaluation

Who refers my child for an evaluation?

Although pediatricians have become more aware of sensory processing disorder and occasionally a teacher may suggest that a child be evaluated, in general, it is a parent who gets the ball rolling. The parents, who spend the most uninterrupted time with their child, are usually well aware of their child's odd behaviors but can't figure out why they are happening.

Will my child's school conduct an evaluation?

If your child is already receiving OT services within his school system, an OT evaluation has probably been performed by the school therapist. If your child is not receiving OT services in school and you'd like him to, directly request an evaluation. An in-school evaluation will most likely focus more closely on issues related to your child functioning in the school environment (e.g., holding a pencil, handwriting, sitting and attending to school-specific tasks) whereas a private OT evaluation will take a more holistic approach to determine what is the underlying reason the child is not participating (sensory, motor, cognitive) related to function in all settings. That said, there are many excellent school occupational therapists who have the background and training in recognition and treatment of a sensory processing disorder. They will be able to develop and carry out an OT program for your child within the school. The program may involve training staff in how to administer specific sensory strategies (deep pressure, heavy work such as erasing the chalkboard, etc.) geared to your child's needs throughout his school day. The school therapist will also be able to provide therapy and address specific sensory needs in her sessions with your child.

If a teacher suspects your child may have SPD and the school OT does not have the time or equipment to evaluate your child, the school OT may approach you, the parents, to pursue a private OT evaluation. A good school therapist is usually eager for any reports or additional information that may help your child within his school environment. Unfortunately, there are also school therapists who do not have enough experience with SPD to be of great help. Many families seek out a private evaluation because they are frustrated that their child's IEP goals include writing his name but the school won't recognize that he is tactilely defensive and refuses to hold a pencil!

What if I want the evaluation done by a private professional?

Private evaluations to determine if a child has a sensory processing disorder are performed by a pediatric occupational therapist (OT). When a child has autism and a possible sensory processing disorder, families will want to seek out an OT who practices using a "sensory-based approach." What does that mean? A sensory-based approach involves observation of the child and incorporating various sensory strategies to help the child regulate and improve his adaptive response to sensory input. Ideally, the OT that you choose to evaluate your child will have post graduate training in assessing sensory integration processes, and experience administering evaluative tools such as the SIPT: Sensory Integration and Praxis Tests. However, if he has not completed this particular training, the ideal therapist should have gained his expertise through coursework which qualifies him to identify sensory processing disorder and implement strategies to treat a child with autism and SPD. The therapist should also have at least two years of experience applying sensory integration techniques within a clinical setting. Mentorship and guidance for a new therapist is usually provided by a therapist who is certified in sensory integration therapy. The therapist should be up to date on current literature and research and be actively involved in professional peer reviews that continue to enhance his understanding of this disability (Smith-Roley, 1999).

Why do I need a therapist trained in a sensory based approach?

All occupational therapists have the knowledge and expertise to work with a wide range of people with disabilities, but many therapists tend to specialize or work with specific populations. Some occupational therapists work with children who have developmental delays, such as those with Down syndrome or cerebral palsy, to name a few. Many OTs focus on treating children and adults who have had a traumatic brain or spinal cord injury, while another group of OTs may have their expertise working with the geriatric and mentally ill populations. OTs who specialize in treating children with sensory processing issues have seen many children with the same type of behaviors and are generally very adept at diagnosing SPD. Their knowledge and experience using sensory strategies (deep pressure, brushing, vestibular input) within a clinic setting make them particularly effective at training families in how to use therapeutic techniques within the home and school.

What is Occupational Therapy?

The American Occupational Therapy Association (AOTA) defines occupational therapy as the "therapeutic use of work, self-care and play activities to increase independent function, enhance development, and prevent disability. It may include adaptation of task or environment to achieve maximum independence and to enhance the quality of life." In simpler terms, occupational therapy looks at how a person is functioning and what "roadblocks" hinder his ability to achieve success with a task. Strategies and activities are then provided to improve his ability to perform activities of daily living (such as dressing, handwriting, play skills, etc.).

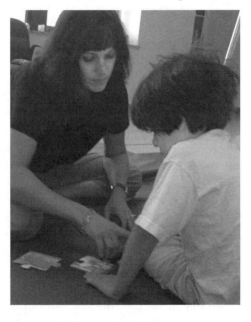

Where can I find an OT to perform the evaluation?

Should you choose to use a private therapist, the first step is to identify a clinic or hospital where you can find an OT who is trained to perform an evaluation with a focus on evaluating sensory processing. An OT who doesn't look at the sensory piece is more likely to assume your child's refusal to eat certain food or hold a pencil is a behavioral issue. The evaluation process will look at how the child functions in everyday activities and daily living skills and determine what is affecting function, i.e., SPD, motor, cognition, attention, etc.

You can begin by locating large children's hospitals within your area. You can also locate various private practice occupational therapists within your area and inquire whether they are pediatric therapists who are trained using a sensory based approach. Another good resource is to touch base with your child's school OT as she may be aware of some specialists within your area.

It is beneficial to choose an OT who has access to a sensory integration gym onsite with swings, bolsters, trampolines, etc. The assessor can then observe your child's response to some of the sensory equipment to determine if he's having either an under- or over-response to sensory input and to actually begin to sort out which types of sensory strategies might help your child calm or alert to sensory input.

Will insurance companies pay for this type of evaluation?

Private insurance will not cover school occupational therapy evaluations; however, insurance benefits vary from policy to policy, so it's worth making a phone call to your insurer. Many insurance companies need a concrete, practical explanation as to why your child needs an occupational therapy evaluation. While it may be difficult to prove there is a medical need for an evaluation, you may be able to claim it as a means to rule out fine motor or visual motor issues affecting your child's current functioning and development.

What do I need to bring or share with the therapist performing my child's evaluation?

The more information you can supply the therapist, the better. Children with autism and SPD may not respond very well to a strange environment, such as the clinic where the evaluation is taking place. Rest assured, most therapists take this into account and are still able to provide a good evaluation, but it is helpful to bring copies of any reports from school or other facilities or professionals (speech, neuropsychologist, and psychiatrist) who have already seen your child. Although not essential, a video of how your child interacts within his home environment is also helpful.

How can I (or should I?) prepare my child for the OT evaluation?

The goal for the therapist is to help your child relax and feel comfortable by giving them time to ease into things and respecting their right to refuse certain types of input. Anything a parent can do to calm their child before they come to the evaluation will be beneficial. If your child feels more relaxed when he knows what to expect, you might briefly describe what the evaluation process will be like. If your child has a special toy or activity that helps him when he is anxious, it may be advantageous to bring it along.

During the Evaluation

What does the evaluation "look like"?

The evaluation usually lasts about one and a half to two hours. Typically, one or both parents accompany their child. The evaluation is conducted in a small, quiet room with limited distractions. The facility may or may not have an onsite sensory integration gym equipped with swings, bolsters, and trampolines, and so forth. If a gym is not available, the therapist will glean information from parent reporting use of simpler tools, such as ball play with the child. There are several components of an occupational therapy evaluation and they are divided into sections listed below:

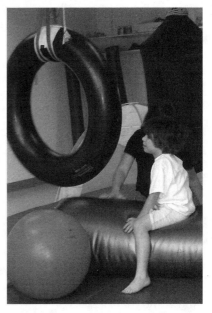

Component #1: Parent Interview. The therapist and parents generally talk first in order to allow the child time to acclimate himself to the new environment and feel as comfortable as possible before interaction with him is begun. Most OTs invite the child to either sit near his parents or explore the room, during which time the therapist is passively observing the child. The interview process is a critical piece of the whole assessment puzzle, given that parents know their child better than anyone else. Telling your family's story provides a wealth of information to the OT, not only about your child's behaviors but how these affect the family as a whole.

What kinds of questions can I expect to be asked?

- The therapist might ask you to describe a typical day for your child. She is trying to determine what is getting in the way of functioning (e.g., refusal to dress, distracted by dangling objects in front of face, screaming in public).
- Can and how much does your child participate with everyday activities (e.g., dressing, feeding)?
- Does your child have any feeding issues (e.g., food refusal, gagging, stuffing food, only eating certain colors or brands)?
- What does your child enjoy doing (e.g., puzzles, playing with the dog)?
- What does your child refuse to do?
- Does he have any self-stimulatory behaviors (e.g., flapping hands, rocking, humming)?
- What behaviors do you think get in the way of your child learning (e.g., humming, refusing to hold objects in hands)?
- What are your goals for your child? What would you like to see your child do (e.g., dress himself, play with a toy, stop biting on everything)?

Component #2: Sensory Histories or Questionnaires. Sensory histories are gleaned from a series of questions asked of parents regarding how their child responds to various types of sensory stimuli. These are very helpful to OTs in that they provide a glimpse into the child's everyday life.

There are many different types of sensory questionnaires. One questionnaire that provides a good source of information about a child's sensory processing system is the Sensory Profile™, developed by Winnie Dunn, Ph.D., OTR, FAOTA. Designed to determine how well children, ages three to ten years, process sensory information in everyday situations, the profile is usually filled out by a parent or caregiver who is familiar with the child. It is arranged into eight categories and has the caregiver answer questions about how the child responds to certain types of sensory input. The results of the profile provide the therapist with some insight into whether the child may be responding in an under- or over-responsive way to various types of sensory input. The scores will place a child in one of three categories:

1) typical performance, i.e., no concerns with sensory issues, 2) possible difference, i.e., some concerns but not something to worry about, 3) definite difference, i.e., lots of sensory issues that may indicate the child is over- or under-responsive to sensory input.

Component #3: Clinical Observations. During this portion of the assessment, the OT gathers information from observing the child, either in free play and/or with use of objects. Reaction to various types of stimuli (swing, trampoline, Sit 'n' Spin, various textured toys, etc.) is observed and reviewed with the family. The tests or activities that an OT might use during the evaluation will most likely depend on your child's age and level of understanding. For example, a child with Asperger's disorder will more than likely be able to communicate and engage in simple reciprocal play activities. Some children will even be able to participate in a formalized fine motor or visual motor test such as the Peabody Fine Motor™ or the Visual Motor Integration™ test. During these tests, the OT will observe the child doing such things as building with blocks, engaging in scissor or pencil skills, and identifying or reproducing shapes. (For those who want more in-depth information about the available formalized tests, a resource section is provided at the back of this book.)

Observation of how the child responds during the testing process is important. Can he remain seated in a chair or does he get up and down? Does he have to "talk himself" through the test (an anxious child sometimes does this to calm himself)? Does he cooperate with directions for all parts of the test or only with some components (e.g., refuses to hold or use a pencil)?

If your child is non-verbal, very anxious, or has limited socialization skills, the OT may observe your child on a floor mat where he can engage in activities that he deems comforting, often self-stimulatory behaviors like dangling beads, perseverating on a familiar toy, rolling on the floor, etc. Since the goal of the evaluation is to find out if your child has a sensory processing disorder, the OT will initiate activities designed to provoke a reaction. An example could be placing play dough in the child's hands if he is tactilely defensive. When the item is placed in the hand, the therapist may try to apply deep pressure, as this is calming and your child may tolerate the play dough for a few seconds more. The therapist is always focused on the child's face and body, looking for a reaction (either alerting or avoidance behavior) as this is a window into your child's sensory profile.

During the clinical observation portion, the therapist is not only trying to determine what sensory-related behaviors your child engages in (e.g., running around the room and banging into the walls), she is also trying to provide possible explanations as to why your child may be doing these things. Is it in response to being in a strange environment? Is it in an effort to avoid the vestibular input from the swing? Does the behavior change or get worse when the child enters the large room with equipment versus the small quiet room? Most of the answers will be assumptions and possibly, as the parent, you will be able to provide additional information about when and where your child does these things at home.

The OT will experiment with some strategies that may help your child calm or alert, such as gentle rocking on a swing, deep pressure to the arms and legs, brushing, or vibration, to try to find "the just right" input that may help your child calm or alert.

Component #4: Parent Training. Other than determining what a child's particular sensory issues are, the second thing an OT does during an evaluation is provide the family with workable strategies and techniques to use with their child at home. The parent training usually begins during the evaluation with the therapist showing and telling what they are doing as they try out various forms of sensory input that may calm, alert, or focus the child. If ongoing occupational therapy is recommended, training will continue with each session as the child's need change. If there is a wait-list for therapy, a follow-up appointment should be scheduled so more training for the parents can be provided.

Areas of Assessment

On pages 63-65 is a chart listing the categories that are evaluated during an occupational therapy assessment and what the therapist does to elicit a sensory response from the child. The third column includes examples of both under- or over-responses to sensory input. The fourth column describes behavior that may be sensory-related but is also often seen in children whose primary diagnosis is ASD.

Keep in mind that this list is just a small sampling of some of the observations that may or may not be observed during the OT evaluation. Every child will "paint" a different picture, and as you can see,

Area of Assessment	Exercise/Activity	Signs of Sensory Dysfunction	Autistic-like Behavior
Gross Motor	OT observes the child using his large muscles to perform activities such as jumping, running, climbing, ball play. Looks at how the child uses balance, posture, strength, and motor planning skills to perform the activities.	Child may avoid any type of movement and cry when asked to sit on a swing with feet off the ground. May run around the room and constantly trip or fall off equipment. May have difficulty keeping his balance.	■ Decreased safety awareness ■ Impulsivity ■ Gets upset if physically moved ■ Excessive jumping, flapping, spinning ■ Crashing, bumping into objects ■ Refusing to ride a bike or use swings, etc.
Fine Motor	OT observes the child's precise fine motor skills, hand grasp, use of both hands to play with a toy, open containers, use markers, activate a toy, etc.	Child may refuse to hold or touch objects. May be interested in a toy but have a limited or lack of fine motor skills to activate or play with a toy. May press too hard or too light with crayons; may break toys by accident.	Child may spin or twirl objects, often within the peripheral visual field (off to the side of the eye), or may refuse to hold objects at all. May mouth toys. May demonstrate inconsistent hand skills (highly skilled for an activity of interest, e.g., drawing with intricate detail but cannot demonstrate same skill with less interesting task, e.g., writing his name).
Oral Motor	OT conducts a history with parent of what the child will eat and, if possible, will observe child's oral motor skills to eat and drink.	Child may only eat certain types of foods (e.g., soft, crunchy, sour). May get upset when texture is added or gag when texture enters his mouth. May stuff his mouth with food or be unaware that food is on his face.	Child may refuse to eat certain food or only eat certain colored (e.g., white) or labeled foods (e.g., Chiquita® bananas). May eat a variety of textures but have major food selectivity (e.g., only eat oranges and spaghetti and meatballs).

(Continued on next page.)

(Continued from previous page.)

Area of Assessment	Exercise/Activity	Signs of Sensory Dysfunction	Autistic-like Behavior
Activities of Daily Living	OT conducts an interview with parent of how child performs dressing, self-feeding, grooming, bathing, and toileting. Depending on the comfort level of the child, may observe dressing and self-feeding.	Family may report that child is a messy eater, doesn't seem aware that his clothes are on backwards, will avoid wearing certain clothing due to feel or smell, refuse to hold a spoon or cup, hate to have teeth brushed, become upset with the sound of toilet flushing, etc.	Family may report that child has toileting training issues related to "holding" his bowels. Child may refuse to participate in dressing or only want to wear red snow boots or a certain T-shirt. May only eat with a certain spoon or plate.
Play Skills	OT observes how the child interacts with toys in the room, looking at motivation, attention, visual focusing, motor planning, cause/effect, interest level, toys of interest.	Child may only want to play with certain toys and doesn't seem to care or know what to do with a new toy. Tends to break all of his toys. May be interested in playing with other children but tends to run around and not have a "game plan." Does not like other children to get too close to him.	Child mostly plays by himself. May have no play skills or interest in toys. May become obsessed with engaging in a repetitive activity. May get upset if another child tries to engage or play with him.
Behavior	OT observes the child's performance with gross motor, fine motor, oral motor, and play skills, and interaction with family, therapist, and room environment. Looks for anxiety, noncompliance,	Child may be calm in a small room but become very "wild," pushing over toys or equipment, in a larger gym. May be upset by noises from another room. May cry or cover his head to therapist's demands. May refuse to	Child may display extreme distress for no apparent reason and may hit himself or others. May become very upset if he is self-stimming on an object and it is removed. May ignore requests to engage in testing or play

	or odd behaviors, possibly in response to types of input (i.e., background noise, toys).	cooperate and prefer to crawl under a desk and rock back and forth.	activity. May be singularly focused on a certain topic, e.g., trains.
Sensory	OT observes child's response to the room (small room vs. large gym), interaction with toys and sensory input (over-responsive or under-responsive). Is he seeking out or avoiding sensory input?	(See above and below.)	■ Teeth-grinding ■ Humming ■ Hand-flapping ■ Staring at lights ■ Rocking ■ Making strange noises ■ Decreased eye contact
Parent/ Child Interaction	OT observes child in response to his family, i.e., avoidance, interaction, what "sets him off"? Looks at whether family "plays into" child's behavior and at parent strategies that are successful and unsuccessful.	Intuitively, a parent may know what calms his child and provide the child with objects that actually increase self-stimming. Child may calm when the parent picks him up and provides deep pressure to his body. Usually during the evaluation, parents are very good at identifying major roadblocks and frustrations that they perceive to be negatively affecting the family unit.	Parent may be very calm, dealing relatively easily with child, or easily distressed and frustrated, feeding into the child's behavior. Parents may also instinctively know what helps their child to calm or alert to a situation.
Parents' Concerns or Goals	OT determines the major areas of concern that affect the child's ability to participate. Acknowledges the parents' issues and goals for their child.	Parents often express frustration with their child's inability to interact within the family routine, and inability to take their child out to "fun" events.	■ Strict adherence to structure and routine. ■ Rigid behavior related to certain foods, clothing, TV shows, play, etc.

to an untrained eye, there is no definite, clear distinction between what is true autistic behavior versus what is a sensory response. An experienced OT with good observation skills will help tease out what is sensory-related behavior and which specific sensory strategies (e.g., tactile activities to increase tolerance, or "heavy work") may help to change some of your child's abnormal behavioral responses that affect his learning and daily functioning. This, along with helping the family identify when and where to provide the needed sensory input, should produce positive changes and improve the child's participation in daily activities. Following is a case study which should give you a clearer picture of an OT evaluation.

Case Study: Marco

Marco is a six-year-old boy who was diagnosed with autism at the age of four. He is currently enrolled in a self-contained classroom at his local public elementary school. The school provides Marco OT services for thirty minutes once a week.

Marco's mom reports that Marco does not dress himself and will not hold a spoon or cup. He eats regular table food but he does not always

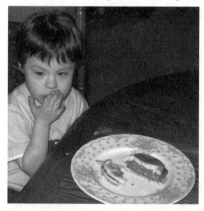

chew up his food and often stuffs too much in his mouth. She is also concerned that he does not play with toys and if he was allowed, would watch TV all day long. When the TV is off, he cannot seem to "entertain himself." He usually runs around the room and often pushes the dining room chairs over. His mother feels he could benefit from more therapy. She has made an appointment at the local hospital for a private OT evaluation in order to determine if Marco needs more therapy than the school is currently offering.

The private session starts out in a small evaluation room. While his mother is being interviewed by the OT, Marco sits on the floor with a bag of toys. The toys that capture Marco's attention are ones that are squishy or balls that have liquid in them. He seems to enjoy pressing them between his hands and pushing them onto the floor. When he tires of this, he runs around the room and locates a large bolster, which he picks up and bangs against the floor. This is removed for fear he might hurt someone or himself. A small trampoline is then brought into the room and Marco happily goes over to jump, but his jumping is very fast and hard. When he steps off the trampoline, he does not appear any calmer. He sits for a few minutes at a small desk, where he is again given some squishy toys. Before long he gets back up and runs around the room. Although the goal is to perform formalized testing, sometimes this is not feasible, so the OT keeps Marco as calm and engaged as she can while she assesses his strengths and weaknesses.

With the interview portion over, Marco's mother asks Marco to sit on the floor while she rubs his head, which she reports he likes. After about a minute, although he doesn't appear angry, Marco pulls hard at his mom's neck and tries to push her over. At that point, the bolster is brought back into the room and as Marco sits on the floor, the therapist rolls the bolster over his legs. He looks up and smiles. He lies on his stomach and lets the therapist roll the bolster over his back. He allows this for about two to three minutes and then is asked to sit at the desk. While at the desk, he again pushes and squeezes the squishy toys and seems to calm down. This time he spends a moment visually inspecting the toys and moves them around in his hands. Since Marco has shown an interest in balls, the therapist rolls one over the desk towards him. He looks at the therapist and rolls it back.

Later in the session, Marco is given some pudding. A spoon is of-fered but he pushes it away. The therapist spoon-feeds him some pudding to get him interested and on the third taste, places Marco's hand on the spoon and provides some deep pressure (therapist's hand on top of Marco's hand). A little resistance is noted but after a few seconds, Marco allows his hand on the spoon and brings it to his mouth. He is also given some cheese curls, which he likes. At first he only bites using his front teeth, but when the thera-

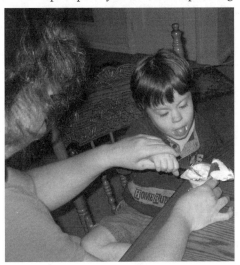

pist scrapes the cheese curl against his molars, he does not resist. When offered another bite, he allows it to be placed on his molars and even does some chewing with his back teeth.

Synopsis

Although this was a short session, many things were determined during this evaluation. Marco appears to be over-responsive to objects placed in his hands, but when he is provided deep pressure (therapist's hand on top of his), he relaxes and calms to this input. Marco seems to be seeking out proprioceptive input as seen when he squeezes small balls, pushes his mother, and bangs the bolster on the floor. This could be his way of trying to calm himself in a strange environment, but is likely also due to under-responsiveness, since we know he also runs around at home and knocks over chairs. Marco is displaying both under-responsive (stuffing food in his mouth, decreased chewing skills) and over-responsive reactions to tactile input (refusing to hold spoon).

Unfortunately, many of the strategies Marco uses either to calm down or stimulate his sensory system are not socially appropriate, get in the way of learning, and could even be dangerous to himself or others. So, we need to provide Marco the deep pressure he seeks in a more suitable manner. We saw that he responded well to having the bolster rolled over his body and that once he had this input, he was able to stay seated in the chair and play with the small tactile balls (which were also providing deep pressure). He was able to sit and tolerate some feeding and even held the spoon with help and deep pressure. When some tactile input (scratching his molar with the cheese curl) was provided, he alerted and showed some increased chewing with his molars. Of course, to see any long-term improvement, these techniques will need to be carried over at home.

Throughout the session, the OT provided Marco's mother with information about her son's behaviors from a sensory point of view. She discussed the use of a sensory diet and showed Marco's mother different types of strategies to try at home, including deep pressure and various tactile activities. It was recommended that the family consider having Marco seen for private OT sessions in addition to services in school. During the weekly sessions, Marco will continue to receive therapy while his mom is further trained in how to provide and maintain an appropriate sensory diet for her son.

After the Evaluation

What will I learn about my child at the end of the OT evaluation?

Although a typical evaluation is only between one and a half to two hours, an experienced therapist should provide you some insight as to whether or not your child has a sensory processing disorder. This will be determined from the parent interview, clinical observations, and the sensory histories or questionnaires. Towards the end of the evaluation, sensory strategies and techniques will be demonstrated to use at home.

Because Marco, from our case study, was unable to sit and tolerate formalized testing, the therapist chose to forgo it. More than likely it would not have provided an accurate picture of his abilities. Focus was instead on how he tolerated various types of sensory input and what seemed to calm or alert his sensory system.

Often, parents have a limited understanding of sensory processing disorder. During the evaluation, the OT will try to familiarize parents with sensory terms and provide possible explanations for their child's behavior. Many therapists provide families with handouts, reading resources, and useful web addresses to give them a better understanding of SPD. If permissible, it's a good idea to videotape the evaluation as there is usually a great deal of information that is shared during the evaluation itself.

How will I receive the evaluation results?

How you are given the evaluation results will depend on where your child is evaluated. More than likely, you will not leave the initial meeting with a written report. On the day of the evaluation, the focus will be on gathering information, observing your child, and training you in intervention strategies. The OT's full written report is completed and usually sent to the family within two to four weeks. You'll want to be sure to fully read the report to be certain you agree with the findings before sending a copy to your child's pediatrician and school.

What if the OT says my child doesn't have an SI problem but I still believe otherwise?

Remember, children with autism demonstrate many behaviors that overlap and sometimes mimic those that result from SPD, i.e., picky eating habits and repetitive behaviors. Although the majority of children on the autism spectrum will have sensory issues, their degree of sensory involvement may not be affecting their ability to participate in daily routines and play. For example, if a child does not have any significant tactile issues related to dressing but adamantly refuses to dress at an age when independent dressing is expected, this is most likely a behavioral-based problem rather than a sensory-based one.

If you've had your child evaluated and you're satisfied that the therapist addressed the major areas of concern discussed in this chapter, but the OT believes your child's issues aren't sensory driven, likely she will encourage you to seek the advice of a behavioral psychologist, who can determine if the behaviors can be extinguished or controlled through use of a behavioral approach. In the end, however, if you have significant doubts about the results you are given, by all means, get a second opinion.

How do I get my child's school to implement the OT's recommendations? How do I get them into my child's IEP (Individualized Education Program)?

If the school and therapists are truly vested in your child, they will usually welcome the additional information and try to incorporate it into your child's school program. You can bring a copy of the private evaluation to share with the school staff to help establish goals for your child's IEP. Presumably, if the evaluation was performed at the school, the school may be more likely to comply with the OT's recommendations. If you do not feel as though the SPD diagnosis or therapeutic recommendations are being taken seriously enough, you can refuse to sign the IEP and challenge this through due process. (See the Bibliography and Recommended Reading List as well as the Resource section at the back of this book for advocacy related books and websites.)

Is it reasonable to think that the school will be able to address all of my child's sensory issues?

For many children who have mild SPD (i.e., manifested as heavy fidgeting or upset with school PA system), school therapies that provide them with specific types of input to either alert or calm them throughout the day may be sufficient. However, if your child comes to the private evaluation with many issues, such as difficulty with dressing and eating, refusing to hold any type of object, severe clumsiness, and poor motor planning skills, it's highly recommended that you consider private OT services to supplement the school services. Your child's school is only able to address issues related to school performance whereas private therapy can address each individual area of concern, along with establishing a sensory diet, and family training.

5 | How Does Sensory Dysfunction Affect My Child?

In Chapter 3 we discussed various abnormal behaviors that may result from a person taking in either too much or too little sensory information. In this chapter, we go deeper and look specifically at how various areas of daily functioning may be affected by sensory processing disorder. Further, we demonstrate how working with an occupational therapist can break down the sensory hurdles that prevent a child from engaging in learning, attention, play, socialization, sleep, and eating.

Learning

Case Study: Diego

Diego loves swings. If he had his way, he would sit on a swing all day long and have someone push him. His family is concerned about this being the one and only activity Diego seems to enjoy. They have tried to get him to play with his toys to no avail. Unfortunately Diego's typical response is to throw his toys and run away.

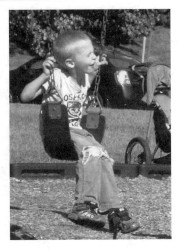

It is very frustrating to try to engage a child who does not want to be engaged. Learning happens when a child is curious and motivated to interact with an object or person or engage in an activity. The activity may be one wherein the child learns through trial and error, such as throwing and catching a ball, or one that someone explicitly teaches him, for example, how to play a board game. It can be difficult to find an activity that will motivate a child with autism to play. It's not hard to see that if Diego is unable to engage or interact—either with objects or people—learning will be stagnated. During therapy, Diego's OT sets up a comforting scenario, looks for windows of opportunity to capture Diego's attention, and then motivates him to engage in an activity. To start, Diego's OT places him on a platform swing in order to give him the sensory input (vestibular) that he craves. However, after the third swing, she stops the movement and asks him if he wants more. He squirms and begins to kick his feet. Even though the OT knows what he is trying to communicate, she does not give in. After about a minute, Diego looks up at her as his way of saying "start the swing" (active participation), and she begins to push the swing. After a few more times, she takes his hands and forms the sign language sign for "more." The demand is now that *he* needs to bring his hands together to try to make the sign. After a minute, his hands come together to form an approximation of the sign and she begins to move the swing.

Neither one of his responses are "miracles." The reason Diego responds is because he likes the sensation of the swing and wants more. Knowing that this is a motivating activity (that he wants to continue)

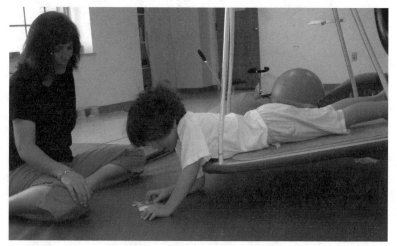

the OT asks Diego to become an active participant. The OT has tapped into the fact that vestibular movement is both enjoyable and alerting to Diego's sensory system and this is where the learning process can begin. Using movement as the motivator, more demands can continue to be placed on Diego, which will help to improve his learning as he continues to enjoy the activity.

Eventually Diego will be expected to take an object and place it in a container, fit a puzzle piece, etc. (all being done while he is on the swing). The activities will eventually become familiar to him, and after a few months he may be able to sit at a desk to complete simple tasks after his body has received some vestibular input. By satisfying Diego's need for vestibular input, which is alerting, his ability to attend to tasks is increased. Determining what motivates Diego and making him an active participant in this process resulted in an increase in his ability to focus and learning could begin.

Attention

Case Study: Kenny

Kenny is a four-year-old child with autism. He comes to his therapy session in a small stroller and becomes very upset if he is removed. Even when he is allowed to remain in the stroller, he often cries when toys are provided and he is asked to play. He refuses to hold anything in his hands and often turns his head to focus on the light on the ceiling.

Kenny is demonstrating an over-responsive reaction both to vestibular and tactile input. He is unable to gain any type of satisfaction from a toy since he is so concerned about the feeling of that toy in his hand. He is not able to focus on a task as his brain and central nervous system is engaged in the "fight or flight" mode. He views both movement and tactile input as aversive and he either becomes upset if demands are placed on him ("fight") or shuts down (looking at light) to avoid the interaction ("flight").

Since Kenny is fearful of movement, his therapist starts the session by meeting him "on his turf," i.e., the stroller. While he sits in the stroller, the OT starts to gently move the stroller back and forth. Kenny does not seem to mind this and actually looks up at the therapist in anticipation of the movement. Kenny enjoys songs that rhyme and this is added to the activity. Once comfortable with this, the therapist slips a large blanket under his bottom and against his back and unhooks the stroller's belt. While she moves the stroller and continues to sing the songs, she pulls him slightly forward with the blanket. Although initially upset, Kenny slowly begins to tolerate the input and again anticipates the action. Finally, Kenny is removed from the stroller and placed snugly inside the blanket. Together, the therapist and Kenny's mother slowly begin to swing him back and forth in the blanket as though in a hammock. Kenny not only appears to enjoy the movement but is beginning to tolerate faster movement. This is the start of helping Kenny get out of the stroller and start to "feel" where his body is in relation to space. The slow, linear, vestibular movement is not only calming but helps him to organize his sensory system and increase his ability to attend and learn from an activity.

Play

Case Study: Kayla

Kayla is playing in the schoolyard during recess time. Although she is running in the midst of her classmates, she is not actually interacting with them. One child comes over and asks her to play tag with

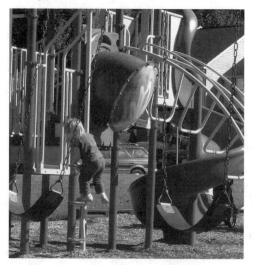

the group. She attempts to join in but trips several times and runs into another child so hard that he falls. After this scenario plays itself out on the playground several times, Kayla's classmates tend to avoid her.

Kayla has poor body awareness in space and has limited motor planning skills. She tries to connect with other children, but she lacks the skills to control her movements and engage appropriately so she can play. Although some of her behaviors are related to her diagnosis of Asperger's disorder, she's also not properly processing incoming sensory information. This prevents her from running and tagging the other children with just the right amount of force. Without the ability to integrate sensory information and form a plan, Kayla runs around the playground fairly aimlessly and without much interaction with the other kids.

Kayla attends weekly OT sessions where she is learning how to improve both her body awareness in space and overall motor planning. Kayla loves to set up obstacle courses using large, foam blocks, fabric tunnels, and bolsters, but often becomes very overwhelmed and pulls out too many objects. She tends to run from one item to the next and when she either falls or doesn't achieve what she wants, she goes to the next item, without truly mastering a task. So, her OT structures a game plan using only two or three items, and gives Kayla regular verbal cues to keep her on task. Kayla provides the motivation and the OT provides the "just right" amount of input that is needed in order for her to "feel" the movement and be successful.

The therapist usually knows when Kayla achieves the "just right" level as she will want to repeat the activity over and over. However, the therapist does not want Kayla to perseverate or get "stuck" on one activity but to be able to use the same action (e.g., balance, movement) in many different situations. To this end, the OT might change the obstacle course set-up. With ongoing therapy, Kayla is beginning to learn what it feels like to move her body in space and by integrating these new skills she should be able to demonstrate more purposeful play skills.

Socialization

Case Study: Michael

Michael is a middle-schooler with Asperger's disorder. A few times a year his family has a big party and all the relatives are invited. Once Michael is aware of the day of the party, he continuously talks about who he is most excited to see and recites stories about some of his favorite uncles. On the day of the party, he gets up early and waits outside for the relatives to arrive. He greets them at the door and seems very pleased that they are

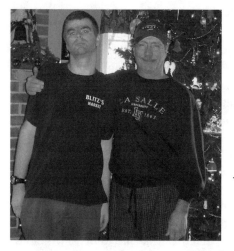

here. However, as more people arrive Michael retreats upstairs to his room and doesn't even come down for dinner. When his mother questions him about why he does not join in, Michael replies that is it too noisy and there are too many smells (perfume, deodorants, fabric softener, etc.).

For children on the autism spectrum, socialization is very difficult, and their attempts to engage with other people can be very awkward. Although this is generally the case with Michael, he feels comfortable with his relatives, who enjoy his company and listen to his stories. Sadly, when the whole family gets together, Michael wants to join in but becomes overwhelmed and unable to filter out all the smells and sounds in order to enjoy the event. While some of us may too feel uneasy in crowds, it's usually not enough to make us leave a party. So, Michael's mother has come up with some strategies to help him. When weather permits, she has the party outdoors where odors may not be as intense. She also provides Michael with soft ear plugs that help muffle some of the extraneous sounds that bother him. In addition, Michael uses his favorite mint flavored lip balm to camouflage the competing odors. Although Michael is still only able to tolerate these events for short periods of time, these strategies allow him to participate and increase his socializations skills.

Sleep

Case Study: Adam

Adam is a four-year-old boy with autism. He attends a preschool program daily and also gets weekly private OT and speech services at a local hospital. He stays pretty active throughout the day and does not take naps. Following his dinner, his mother tries to provide a routine to prepare him for bed. This includes a warm bath, reading favorite stories, and listening *to calming music. Once in bed, though, he tosses and turns and begins to cry. Nothing seems to work except having his mother lie beside him with her arm over him until he finally falls asleep (sometimes not until eleven o'clock). She notes that the later Adam falls asleep, the more "out of it" he is the following day. The routine is beginning to wear on the entire family and Adam's mother admits to his OT that she is running out of patience.*

Anyone who has ever tried to coax an overtired infant to sleep is well aware of the anxiety and frustration this can cause. When children are very young, a parent will often need to go into the child's room numerous times until he settles down. Usually after a few days or weeks, the child learns how to calm and fall asleep on his own. Given that Adam is already four years old and still having trouble falling asleep on his own, it's not hard to see how this current arrangement is negatively affecting Adam's entire family.

Adam's OT feels that Adam has a sensory modulation problem. She confirms that many of the techniques Adam's mom is using are right on target, but that Adam may simply need more. During his OT sessions, she notices that Adam responds well to deep pressure. She recommends the family purchase a large body pillow and fill it with dry beans to weigh it down. When Adam's mother puts him in bed, instead of lying beside him, she is to wedge the pillow against his body where she used to lay. At the OT's suggestion, she covers him with a heavy blanket and tucks him in very tightly. She then reads him a few stories and continues to play soft, calming music in the background. After performing the same routine for about a week, she notices that when she kisses Adam goodnight and leaves the room, he is not getting out of bed. Although there is some whimpering, he usually falls off to sleep within fifteen minutes. Research has shown that deep pressure from pillows can be an effective way to help decrease one's arousal level (Williams & Shellenberger, 1996).

Eating

Case Study: Kenny

Kenny, from our earlier case study, is tall but underweight for his age. He does not have any specific oral motor concerns (difficulty with chewing or swallowing food safely) but is very adamant regarding what types of food he will eat. He likes chicken nuggets but will only eat them after picking off all of the coating. He will eat potato chips and crackers, Cheerios without milk, pasta without sauce, and the rest of the foods he prefers are mostly smooth (e.g., yogurt, pudding, ice cream). If his family tries to encourage him to eat what is being served for dinner, he usually screams and kicks, and mealtime becomes un-pleasant for everyone at the table. Although his mother is concerned about his selective eating habits, she feeds him what she knows he will eat since she wants him to continue to gain weight and grow.

Kenny has tactile issues related to eating. While he eats different textures—both smooth and crunchy—he becomes upset if two textures are in his mouth at the same time (e.g., soft chicken meat and crispy coating). His sensory system cannot handle that much information and is displaying an over-response to the input from the food. Children with autism often have issues related to feeding, which can be similar to Kenny's, or different, i.e., they may only want to eat a certain colored food or items with certain brand names. These types of behaviors are most likely related to the diagnosis of autism. If a food aversion is caused by a sensory problem, there is a good chance the child may be able to slowly learn to increase tolerance for textures or food choices.

Because the OT knows that Kenny (from our earlier case study) is most comfortable in his stroller, she allows him to remain there while she offers him a food that he likes—yogurt. He is given two or three spoonfuls and truly seems to enjoy the taste. His therapist takes a portion of the yogurt and crushes very tiny crumbs of Cheerios into it. Kenny is provided the next spoonful with this mixture and eats it. He is aware of the texture, and although he gags slightly, he swallows the food. The OT then gives him two or three more spoonfuls of the plain yogurt, which he readily accepts. When she again attempts the Cheerio-yogurt mixture, he tolerates two spoonfuls before he realizes that there is something different. She then goes back to the plain yogurt.

The therapist trains Kenny's mom in this strategy and reminds her to observe and respect Kenny's behavioral responses. To see true progress will likely take a great deal of time and daily practice. The goal is for Kenny to not only accept two mixed textures but to gradu-ally increase the size of pieces that are added to the mixture until he is able to tolerate and eat higher level foods.

Impact on Daily Functioning—Home, School, and Community

As we can see from the case studies above, a poor sensory processing system will affect all areas of daily living. Below are two charts which further illustrate this point. The first chart illustrates the impact for a child, such as Kenny, who presents with an over-responsive sensory system, while the second chart portrays a child, like Kayla, with an under-responsive sensory system. Keep in mind that both children have been diagnosed on the autistic spectrum *and* have a sensory processing disorder.

Conclusion

As parents, our goal is to keep our children safe and help them grow up to be as independent as they can possibly be. For parents of children with autism, this can be especially difficult. Add to that a sensory processing disorder and you've got a real challenge on your hands. One that will require your patience and skills and the knowledge and support of various professionals. As you explore the next few chapters of this book, hopefully you will find strategies and techniques that will help to improve your child's ability to process sensory information more effectively and increase his level of independence with everyday living skills.

Over-Responsive Sensory System

Sensory System	Function	Impact
Tactile Views all tactile (touch) information as harmful. Usually responds with crying, anxiety, or avoidance. Noted in a child's decreased ability to hold onto everyday items, difficulty with wearing clothing, having face washed, and teeth brushed.	**Fine Motor** ■ Dressing ■ Grooming ■ Self-feeding	The child refuses to hold items in his hands, which affects his ability to learn how to manipulate clothes, fasteners, toothbrushes, feeding utensils, etc. As the child gets older and bigger, more independence in daily skills is expected. When this does not happen, the child's family becomes more put upon and can become frustrated.
	■ Play ■ Preschool tasks, e.g., coloring, cutting, gluing	The child typically becomes upset if other children touch him or get close to him. He avoids activities that involve use of his hands, e.g., play or preschool tasks, and may become disruptive, e.g., screaming or lashing out when such demands are placed on him. This affects the child's ability to learn how to draw, write his name, manipulate objects, etc.
	Oral Motor Eating – including appropriate participation and eating skills at mealtimes in various settings	Due to the child's hypersensitivity to texture, he will only eat certain foods and avoids the majority of food choices. This can affect the child's energy level, ability to attend, as well as overall growth and nutritional health.
■ Picky eater ■ Avoids having two textures in mouth at the same time ■ Odd eating habits		

■ Avoids or gets upset with circle time ■ Stays by himself on the playground ■ Does not join in peer play activities, such as ball games	**Gross Motor** ■ Balance ■ Endurance ■ Strength	Child may not want to interact in gross motor games such as tag or Follow the Leader due to his concern about being touched.
Vestibular The child views any type of movement as anxiety-provoking. Tends to stay in one spot as he has difficulty processing the impact of gravity on his system.	**Movement** ■ Playground activities ■ Sports ■ Group play with peers	The child tends to stay in one spot and, when moved, will most likely cry and become very upset, especially if his feet are not touching the ground. He does not seek out activities that involve movement, as his vestibular system cannot process the impact of gravity on his body and he experiences it as frightening.
Proprioceptive The child does not experience and learn from movement due to his fear of it.	**Body Awareness** ■ Playing ball games (catch, soccer, etc.) ■ Climbing ■ Motor planning involved in self-feeding and dressing	Because the child has a fear of movement and an inability to feel where his body is in relation to space, he does not experience new body patterns or activities. This results in poor motor planning skills.
Auditory The child experiences oversensitivity to sounds. He has difficulty processing all types of sounds.	**Socialization** ■ Participating in school circle time ■ Playing games with peers ■ Participating in "fun" activities like parties, family meals, circus, etc.	He cannot handle too many sounds and tends to block out the majority of sounds entering his brain either by plugging his ears or shouting or crying over the noise. Because he is unable to process auditory information, he has difficulty responding to questions or interacting with people.

Under-Responsive Sensory System

Sensory System	Function	Impact
Tactile The child tends to go around touching everything but has a great deal of difficulty processing the tactile input to gather the just right amount of information that is needed to perform a task.	**Fine Motor** ■ Dressing ■ Grooming ■ Self-feeding	The child tends to put clothes on backwards without realizing the mistake. Has difficulty with fasteners and has a weak grasp to hold utensils or brush teeth.
	■ Play ■ School tasks, e.g., coloring, cutting, gluing, handwriting	Does not know boundaries. Gets too close to other children and tends to play too rough. Difficulty with holding a pencil, using scissors, keeping letters on the line.
	Oral Motor Eating – including appropriate participation and eating skills at mealtimes in various settings	Eats with fingers, stuffs food in mouth, chews with open mouth, doesn't seem aware of being messy

MIXED SIGNALS | 85

 ■ Engages in rough play ■ Does not seem to know his own strength and may hurt another child ■ Falls often or is very clumsy ■ Has difficulty with ball activities, i.e., throws either too hard or too soft	**Gross Motor** ■ Balance ■ Endurance ■ Strength	■ Tactile sensory issues affect child's body awareness to interact and play gross motor games effectively ■ Other children tend to avoid this child for fear of getting hurt
Vestibular	**Movement** ■ Group activities with rules ■ Playground activities ■ Safety awareness	Child craves a lot of movement and usually does not know when to stop. Tends to be disruptive as he has difficulty following instructions, playing a game, taking turns.
Proprioceptive	**Body Awareness** ■ Navigating school hallways and cafeteria ■ Playing ball games (catch, soccer, etc.) ■ Craft projects ■ Meal preparation (making a sandwich, pouring juice) ■ Motor planning involved in self-feeding and dressing	The child has poor motor planning skills due to the fact that he is not processing "how much" or "how little" pressure needs to be applied to hold a pencil, tag another child, throw or catch a ball. Presents as clumsy and awkward.
Auditory	**Socialization** ■ Developing friendships ■ Taking turns ■ Reading body language and physical cues	Child does not know how to regulate voice volume and is typically either too loud or too quiet.

6 Is Sensory Integration Therapy Right for My Child?

The objective of therapy using a sensory integrative approach for the child with autism is to improve sensory processing so that more sensations will be effectively "registered" and modulated, and to encourage the child to form simple adaptive responses as a means of helping him to learn to organize his behavior. When this type of therapy does make a difference, the child's life is changed considerably; but at this time, no therapy can "cure" autism.

—Jean Ayres, 1979

Remember Kenny? The four-year-old child with autism who didn't want to venture out of his stroller? Kenny has been receiving OT services for the past six months. Today he is attending his weekly OT session at a local hospital.

Sitting on a large platform swing, Kenny looks up at his therapist, prompting her to push the swing. She does so and Kenny laughs and makes soft guttural noises. When the swing stops, he again looks at the OT and signs the word "more." She pushes the swing at his request. After a few minutes the swing stops and the therapist gives Kenny a ball of playdough. He takes it readily and pushes it into his hands. The therapist helps him push the playdough onto a flat surface and then gives him a small cookie cutter to push into the dough. At first, Kenny resists the invitation as he just wants to squeeze the playdough. But with gentle insistence, he holds the cutter, as it is guided into the playdough.

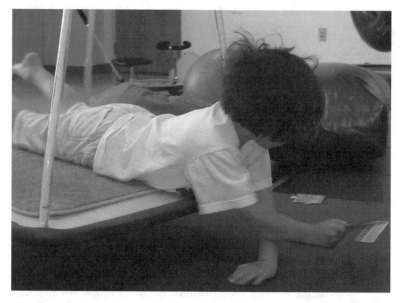

The therapist removes the cookie cutter and Kenny sees an image of the shape. He quickly picks up the shape and reforms it into a blob, starting the process all over again.

To the reader, what has taken place during this occupational therapy session may not seem all that special, but to Kenny's mother, it is monumental. Six months ago, Kenny was very fearful of any type of movement and would scream if he was removed from his stroller. He became very upset if anything was placed even near his hands. Any type of sensory activity needed to be introduced through his feet, which were not as tactilely defensive as his hands. For example, the occupational therapist first placed playdough against the bottom of Kenny's feet using deep pressure. (This type of input helped calm and organize his sensory system so he could accept the tactile input.)

During the early days of therapy, Kenny did not sign or engage in eye contact. Now, even though his signs and eye contact are limited, Kenny will look at the therapist and use some signs when an activity is of interest to him and he wants it to continue. While Kenny continues to be fearful of new types of movement (e.g., Sit 'n' Spin), once it is introduced through the use of deep pressure and a slow, consistent force, he not only accepts, but actually appears to crave the vestibular input.

What Does an Occupational Therapist Do?

The therapy that Kenny is receiving is performed by an occupational therapist (OT) who is trained in the use of a sensory-based approach. OTs practice in various settings including hospitals, schools, nursing homes, workshops, or in private practice settings. They often work with elderly people or with people with disabilities (either from birth or acquired, such as a head or spinal cord injury). The goal of any occupational therapist is to improve his clients' ability to be independent and to help provide meaning and purpose to daily activities. This includes any task performed at work, play, or in the community. In this context, daily activities not only include practical tasks such as dressing or grooming but really any action or activity that is important to an individual, such as playing catch with a friend, or independently making mac'n'cheese in the microwave.

Occupational therapists begin by observing their clients in play or while performing a task so as to determine strengths and weaknesses. They try to break down the areas of difficulty that may be preventing a person from actively participating in an activity. After analyzing the information, they provide strategies or adaptations that will enable that person to be successful with performance of a daily activity. These techniques help the person slowly increase his skill level, which in turn builds his confidence and motivation to engage in tasks.

Occupational therapists typically attend a four-year academic program. Upon fulfilling all of the requirements set up by the American Occupational Therapy Association (AOTA) including two separate three-month-long affiliations (generally one in mental health, the other in physical disabilities), six months of supervised fieldwork, licensing, and passing a four-hour certification test, they are registered to practice occupational therapy. To maintain licensure, all OTs must provide proof of continuing education or professional development. Most therapists fulfill this requirement by taking coursework in areas of specific interest to them (e.g., feeding and swallowing or hand deformities).

What is a "Sensory-Based Approach" to Occupational Therapy?

Occupational therapists tend to find their niche and focus on working with specific populations (e.g., adults, children). Many OTs who opt to work with the pediatric population have discovered that using a sensory integrative treatment approach appears to work well with children diagnosed with AD/HD (attention deficit/hyperactivity disorder), LD (learning disabilities), and autism. A sensory-based approach involves use of sensory enriched activities, such as swings, therapy balls, and trampolines. The focus is on providing the child opportunities to experience sensation at just the right level for his particular system. OTs who are experienced in the use of sensory integration therapy use play—a child's primary occupation—as a means to identify and address many of the behaviors the child may be exhibiting (over- or under-responses) to various types of sensory input. She studies the abnormal affect these responses have on a child's daily functioning in play, socialization, eating, dressing, etc. Through use of various sensory techniques (e.g., gym equipment, deep pressure) the therapist provides the child with the "just right" amount of sensory input that he can tolerate, along with engaging him in sensory activities that will help calm or alert him. By using this approach, the child begins to accept and respond more appropriately to play and daily activities. (In-depth explanation of specific treatment techniques will be described in Chapter 7.)

Within a certified school program, all OTs receive some basic background in sensory integration theory; however, the majority of therapists who choose to pursue this specific avenue further their training through graduate programs or lengthy seminars in sensory integration theory and treatment. These seminars are usually conducted by seasoned OTs along with professionals of various other disciplines, such as psychologists, physicians, and teachers, who are currently involved in ongoing research that is beginning to demonstrate the positive effect of diagnosing and treating SPD.

How Will This Type of Therapy Help My Child?

Looking at Kenny as our example, we begin to understand how a sensory based approach works for children with sensory processing disorder. In the case study above, Kenny had been attending private speech and occupational therapy for about a year. But during his initial OT sessions, any type of input (deep pressure, brushing) was always introduced while Kenny sat in his stroller. The therapist constantly observed Kenny's response to sensory input. When Kenny was offered any type of toy to hold, his eyes would widen and his fingers would spread very far apart. He not only refused to touch the item, but would usually turn his head and kick his feet against the side of his stroller.

During early sessions, the therapist noted that Kenny always wanted his shoes off, so she began to press objects to the bottoms of his feet. To this, Kenny would look up and smile. On a few occasions, he would bring his foot up to the therapist. This act of bringing his foot up for more interaction was Kenny's first adaptive response. (His feet were not as tactilely defensive as his hands and he actually liked the input.) Slowly, the input that he tolerated to his feet was provided to his hands, along with lots of deep pressure. If Kenny became upset, the input was stopped for a few seconds. Once he calmed, the input was shown to him and tried again. Gradually, Kenny began to hold a stress ball and eventually playdough for brief periods of time. He was finally beginning to tolerate some tactile input to his hands.

Typically, we use our various senses (hearing, touch, vision, etc.) to not only gather sensory information from an object but to gradually integrate all the information in order to learn how to play with or use that object. Tolerating input—looking for that "just right" level—is how we learn to modulate our sensory system. But Kenny has a sensory modulation disorder, a subgroup of sensory processing disorder. As a result, he avoids the input (sensory avoiding) with consequences noted in his inability to use his hands effectively to play or do everyday activities, such as feeding or dressing himself. Due to his poor sensory processing, Kenny is unable to seek out the sensory information that he needs and that will allow him to tolerate sensation and begin to explore and use his hands. However, with on-going OT, he is slowly beginning to find the "just right" level that he can tolerate and is making progress with his ability to use his hands for everyday tasks, including signing, holding a spoon, and playing with a toy.

Jasmine, the five-year-old girl with Asperger's disorder who was introduced in Chapter 3, also demonstrates a sensory modulation disorder. She is always seeking out sensory input but is unable to register the sensory information adequately in order to continue to improve her clumsiness and poor motor planning skills. She has been attending weekly OT sessions for the past six months and we can see how the sensory based approach is helping her with SPD.

During therapy sessions, Jasmine usually enters the room and runs from one piece of gym equipment to the next. She does not seem to have a game plan regarding how to use the apparatus so she runs around the room or demands other pieces of equipment. The therapist helps Jasmine pick out a large, foam-filled pillow, which Jasmine immediately dives into, laughing and getting sillier and sillier. The therapist takes Jasmine's hand and tells her to imagine the pillow is a large cloud in the sky. Her task is to try to climb to the top in order to look down at the world. The deep pressure from the pillow helps Jasmine get organized and, as she tries repeatedly to climb up the "cloud," the effort produced provides "heavy work." Jasmine remains very focused. With each trial, the therapist provides her a little more tactile input (offering hands to help her pull up) and by the fourth attempt, Jasmine reaches the top and wants to do it again. Each time she succeeds a little quicker than the last time.

Settled at the top of the pillow, the therapist tells Jasmine to look down at the floor, where there are toy fish. They make-believe she is hungry and needs to catch some fish to eat. Jasmine is provided with a

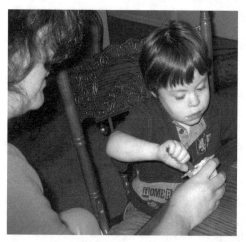

long fishing rod that can touch the floor. Instead of staying on the top of the cloud, Jasmine slides off to get closer to the floor. The therapist encourages her to go back to the top where she will hold Jasmine at her waist (deep pressure) as she leans forward to "catch" the fish. The first few times, Jasmine leans too far forward and almost loses her balance. But with each trial, the therapist gives her a little more input and guidance (of where her body is in space) as she leans forward to catch a fish. She finally catches a fish and is very happy. She wants to repeat the activity and with each try, she begins to know just how far she needs to reach out to catch the fish without losing her balance. As Jasmine's skills and body awareness improve, she is able to keep her balance and the therapist no longer needs to hold her.

This may seem like simple child's play, but in reality, it is just the opposite. Jasmine does not have the skills to play appropriately and needs to learn them. These OT activities allowed Jasmine to play and use her imagination to set up a story while she worked on developing balance and motor planning skills. The activity helped her to gain the "just right" amount of sensory information, which was required to enjoy her adventure and motivate her to continue in play.

All children have an inner drive to satisfy their needs, those needs just may be a bit harder to identify in your child. A sensory-based therapy approach can help your child achieve the "just right" amount of stimulation, and the strategies introduced will likely prove to be more socially acceptable than your child's previous attempts to manage his sensory needs (e.g., aimlessly running around the room, refusing to hold objects). Through daily structure and ongoing parent training in the use of many of the sensory-based strategies, your child should begin to improve his ability to dress, self-feed, tolerate various types of input, and participate in a more typical family routine.

What Are the Long-Term Effects of Not Processing Sensory Information Effectively?

Each child in the scenarios above presents with a totally different picture; however, with the right type of sensory approach, both benefit from their specialized occupational therapy services. Therapy is a long-term process and sensory information must be pro-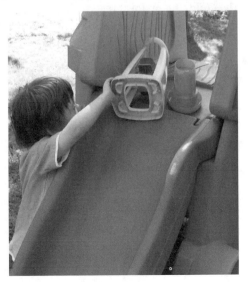vided at the level where your child is both comfortable and accepting of it in order to produce the adaptive response needed for processing and learning. Before therapy, Kenny wanted to stay in his stroller where he felt safe, despite the fact that he could walk. Staying in that "safe" environment prevents him from interacting with the rest of the world. You can imagine how much more impaired Kenny would be if he was unwilling to tolerate sensory input. Through therapy, Kenny has learned to use his hands for playing, feeding, dressing, as well as signing to communicate.

Jasmine, on the other hand, while verbal, is clumsy, is very disorganized when it comes to play. She wants to fit in with other children, but is unable to play appropriately; her silliness and rambunctious behavior tends to get her in trouble. Through occupational therapy, Jasmine now has a better chance to learn where her body is in space and how to use it more effectively for game-playing and interacting with other children. Using a sensory based treatment approach will not cure either one of these children but it will begin to help them process sensory information more effectively so they can play and interact with their world.

Can This Type of Therapy Be Harmful to My Child?

The answer to this question is no, provided therapy is done by an accredited occupational therapist, experienced in working with children diagnosed with SPD. Although to the untrained eye this type of therapy may just look like play, the therapist is always observing the child's behavioral responses to sensory input. She will know how much sensory input the child can handle and when it is time to offer him more or give the child a rest.

Be aware that determining a child's sensory needs is not always intuitive. For example, a child who appears lethargic and presents as being under-responsive may in fact be extremely over-responsive—so fearful of movement or touch that he enters a shut down mode (the central nervous system's "flight" response). An untrained or inexperienced OT may attempt techniques aimed at alerting this child's system and inadvertently do more harm than good. An astute therapist trained in a sensory based approach can recognize this child's bodily reactions and determine the appropriate, therapeutic approach that will help increase his level of tolerance and function.

Although your child may be fearful or initially avoid sensory input, the experienced therapist can determine how much is too much. A trained OT will use a slow, gradual approach and to continue to up the ante—making more demands in order to increase the child's active participation and use of appropriate strategies to engage in daily tasks. Generally, most kids view therapy as a fun and safe activity. While the therapist alone cannot provide the optimal amount of input to meet your child's sensory diet needs, she will train you to read your child's behavioral signs and apply the appropriate techniques to provide your child the right amount of sensory input on a daily basis.

How Do I Know If this Approach Will Work for My Child?

Therapists have been using many of the sensory strategies for many years. Although parents, therapists, and, often, the children are able to tell you it works, that alone should not be enough to convince you. Research is actively being done in order to prove the effectiveness of use of a sensory based approach. A list of books detailing current research can be found at the end of this book, but below is a list of some of the results that have been documented to justify the claims of using a sensory based approach on a child with autism.

- Deep pressure input appears to have a calming effect on behavior (increased social interaction and attention). (Edelson, Edelson, Kerr, and Grandin, 1999).
- Use of sensory techniques was documented to be more effective on children with autism with over-aroused responses to sensory input. (Ayres, Tickel, 1980).
- Decreased self-injurious behaviors and an increase in purposeful activities and socialization following short sessions of planned sensory input on a daily basis. (Larrington, 1987: Lemke, 1974: McClure & Holtz-Yotz,1991: Reisman, 1993)

Can a Sensory Diet Stop My Child From Engaging in Unwanted and Self-Injurious Behaviors?

Yes, a sensory diet can help extinguish unwanted behavior as long as the reason the child is engaging in the behavior is to get more sensory input. Take, for example, a child who sucks and chews on his fingers until they are raw and cracked (putting him at risk for infection). His tactile responses are so low that in order to "feel" his fingers, he needs to feel pain. An OT might recommend a brushing program and the use of small squeeze toys that provide deep pressure. Often a behavior, such as this, may develop due to a sensory need but evolve into an obsessive behavior. Even though your child may begin to respond to the sensory input (deep pressure and brushing), he may still sometimes engage in this abnormal behavior. You will need to be patient and slowly begin to substitute the more "normal" behavior through sensory input (brushing and squeeze toys) when your child wants to continue with the old behavior (fingers in the mouth). With patience and persistence, hopefully your child will find that he is getting the "right" type of input from the substitute and allow it to replace the unwanted behavior.

What is the Ultimate Goal of a Sensory Integration Treatment Approach?

Children with a SPD will most likely always have issues with their ability to process sensory information effectively, but the appropriate therapy can affect the degree to which their lives are affected. The goal of using this type of treatment is to provide various sensory strategies to help the child improve tolerance and understanding of

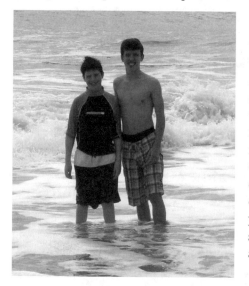

incoming sensory input. Using various therapeutic techniques, your child will be more alert and comfortable with sensory input and the focus will shift to using the information more effectively with fine motor and play activities. Once your child's immediate sensory processing concerns are managed, you can focus on teaching skills and addressing his autistic behaviors.

What Happens During Therapy?

Occupational therapy takes a team approach. The team consists of the occupational therapist as the coach, and you, the parents, and your child as players. The OT that's right for your family should view and treat your child as a whole person—not just a set of challenges. An experienced OT will look for areas of strength in your child and use them to tap into his inner drive. From the very first meeting, your OT should attempt to make your child feel comfortable by limiting demands 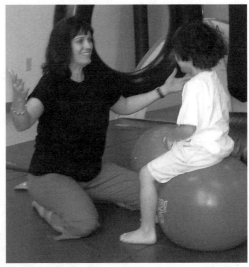 and giving him time to adjust to his new surroundings. She ought to treat you as the number one expert on your child and be willing to listen to your concerns and frustrations. (See Chapter 4 for more detailed information about choosing an OT to conduct your child's evaluation and therapy.)

How Do I Find a Therapist Who Practices a Sensory-Based Approach?

It is essential that you select a therapist who is knowledgeable in working with children diagnosed with SPD. There are many types of therapists who have excellent knowledge of treatment approaches (rehabilitation, hand therapy, school based, etc.) but they will be of no value to your child if they are unable to "tap into" his sensory system before asking him to engage in a daily activity. In order to find this type of therapist, you may want to contact your local children's hospital, touch base with a school therapist, search the Internet, or contact AOTA (American Occupational Therapy Association) or Sensory Integration International for a list of qualified therapists. (Further information is provided in the Resource section at the back of this book.) A very simple and often common avenue is to talk to another parent who has a child with autism or SPD. They may end up being your best resource as they will more than likely have the same or similar goals for their child as you have for your child. They will be able to talk about their own experiences and how sensory-based occupational therapy has helped their child.

Where is Therapy Conducted?

Private therapy is usually provided in a large clinic area that is set up like a gym with many pieces of equipment, for example platform swings, large bolsters, a ball pit, scooters, ramps, large therapy balls, and small trampoline. (A broader discussion of tools and treatment strategies can be found in Chapter 8.) It is set up to appeal to young children, to draw them into the space. However, during the first few sessions your child may be anxious, want to stay close to you, and avoid contact with any of the equipment. If

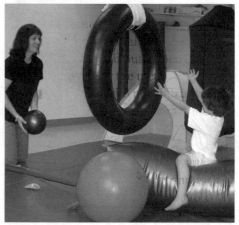

your child is over-responsive, this type of area may be overstimulating. In this case, most clinics have a quiet area where your child may initially be the most comfortable. That area may have a beanbag chair, soft music playing, dimmed lights, books, and maybe some plush toys and blankets. Therapy might be conducted in the quiet area initially until your child feels more comfortable to venture towards the gym equipment.

What Happens During Therapy?

Therapy usually involves the therapist trying out various types of techniques (listed in Chapter 8) to determine what works and what doesn't, although an experienced therapist will probably already have an indication of what types of techniques will work best for your child based on his evaluation. It is important to recognize, however, that although children may share a diagnosis or some common characteristics, no two children are exactly alike. A well trained therapist will be very observant of your child's particular needs and will usually begin very slowly, trying to establish a rap-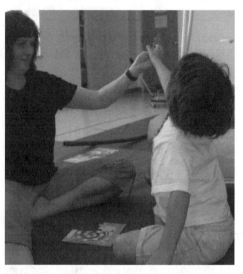port and make up a specific game plan for your child. With each session, more information from both observation and your verbal input will continue to help develop a picture of what types of activities will work best for your child, both in the clinic and at home.

Ideally, a parent should be present during therapy sessions so he can watch how his child reacts to the various types of input. However, some children who are easily distracted or somewhat dependent on their parents may work better if their parent is not in the room. In this case, a parent may be able to observe through a one-way mirror. If this is not possible, the last five to ten minutes of the sessions should be set aside to review techniques and strategies that can be carried over to home.

The therapy environment should be pleasant and motivating to your child. Sessions are "child driven," meaning the OT will follow the child's lead and allow him to choose the activity, which may be as complicated as setting up an obstacle course or as simple as finding a preferred item buried in sand. The role of the OT is to structure the environment such that your child feels at ease, especially as more challenging activities are presented. A good therapy session, from the eyes of an observer, should look like play, when, in fact, it is hard work. The goal of the therapist is to provide the child controlled, or "just right," amounts of sensory input in order to elicit an adaptive response and take the skills to a more functional level.

What If My Child Refuses to Participate? Should I Force Him To Do the Activities?

No. Forcing should never be part of a child's OT session or carry-over therapy at home. However, many children with sensory avoiding behaviors will not seek out sensory input and they will need to be very slowly introduced to steady doses of input until they are comfortable enough to tolerate increasing amounts. Your child's OT will usually be the first one to determine how much is enough, especially for a child who is hypersensitive. She will teach you techniques and give you guidelines as to how to slowly increase the input. Remember, your child may initially whimper or avoid, but should never be screaming or crying. Even children who are over-responsive to sensory input will usually enjoy all the sensory strategies because they should be providing them with sensory input that their systems need at the right dosage that they can handle.

How Should Therapy Goals Be Set?

Goals that will be addressed during the weekly sessions are determined in two ways. First they will be developed from the results of the sensory profile and clinical observations (information that was obtained during the initial evaluation). A goal may be to decrease tactile over-responsivity to the hands or to improve the child's motor planning skills to use a pencil. Secondly, goals are gleaned from the parent interview or specific concerns that have been expressed by the family. For example, a parent's goal may be that his child learns to tolerate getting dressed or using a spoon to eat. Another parent's goal may be to have his child increase his play skills, or be able to remain calm while out in public.

Goals will reflect what the major concerns are for that particular family. It is important for the therapist to listen to the family's concerns and include their particular areas of concern in the goals. Goals will be formally written up and reviewed with the parents. Progress will be documented in weekly notes shared with the family and once set goals are achieved, the process will begin again.

If a goal is unrealistic, many short-term goals will need to be achieved towards the final goal. For example, Amelia's dad may want Amelia to write her name even though she cannot tolerate holding a pencil. The therapist should explain that although the goal is not impossible, there are many short-term goals that need to be met first. Initially, Amelia will be encouraged to explore textured items (e.g., sand, rice, or beans) in 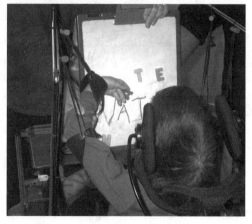 order to increase her tolerance. Then, she may be asked to draw lines in the sand. As her comfort level with textures increases, they'll move on to more functional goals, such as holding a marker, and so on.

Will My Child's Sensory Needs and Goals Change Periodically?

Treatment and goals will change constantly because the objective of therapy is to continually "up the ante" once a skill or activity has been mastered. This is akin to the process of a child just learning to

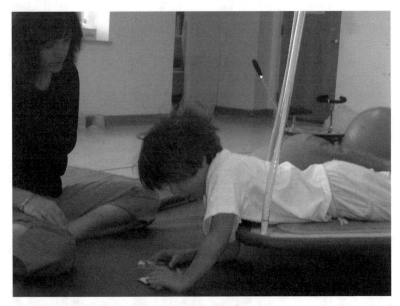

stand who will soon begin walking and then try running, climbing, and jumping in order to keep placing higher level demands on his sensory system to continue to improve his gross motor skills. However, children with a sensory processing disorder do not always know when to up the ante so it becomes the job of the therapist to determine when the activities needs to be changed or made more challenging. For example, your child may initially be very fearful of sitting on a swing, but after repeated exposure will begin to accept the movement. This is the time the OT will encourage him to reach out to grab a beanbag while he is swinging and throw it at a target. The treatment will continually change in this way, depending on how well your child can tolerate or master the current level of sensory input.

Can Private Therapy Goals Be Included In An IEP?

Including goals in the IEP (Individual Education Program) cannot usually be done by a private OT but you, as a parent, can either provide the school a copy of the OT's report or request that your child's private OT go to or phone into an IEP meeting and have her tell the IEP team why your child needs therapy. (Keep in mind that insurance may not cover the expense of your OT's time in a case like this.) If you can prove that your child's OT problems have an educational impact on his abilities to succeed at school and can demonstrate that sensory strategies are working to reduce problematic behavior,

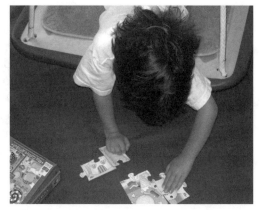

your child's school team should be willing to incorporate therapy at school. If you do not feel as though the SPD diagnosis or therapeutic recommendations are being taken seriously enough, you can refuse to sign the IEP and challenge this through due process. (See the Bibliography and Recommended Reading List as well as the Resource section at the back of this book for advocacy related books and websites.)

How Often Should My Child Attend Therapy Sessions?

Ideally, your child should attend sessions at least once a week, but in today's world and especially with the ever-changing healthcare picture, insurance may not cover weekly sessions. If that is the case, you may attend a few sessions and be trained in use of techniques and strategies that you can carryover at home. A monthly follow-up session is a good idea to re-evaluate and update treatment strategies. Generally, the first five to ten minutes of each therapy session should be devoted to review how therapy is going and to address parents' concerns and questions. It is also beneficial to keep a journal of times and events where therapy approaches appear to be working for your child or not.

How Will I Know If Therapy Is Working Or Not?

Children for whom therapy is working should show marked improvement in attention, body awareness, motor planning skills, and participation in activities of daily living, as well as greater tolerance of sensory input, a decrease in self-stimulatory behaviors, increased food and play repertoire, and so on. Unfortunately, there are some children for whom this type of therapy is not successful. A child may have other areas of concern related more to autism than sensory dysfunction, a component of autism. This will be determined by the therapist following at least six sessions with ongoing carryover at home. However, the majority of children, even those very profoundly affected by autism and sensory issues, will usually demonstrate a positive response to this treatment approach.

8 Treatment Approaches

No one can organize a child's brain for him. He has to do it himself, but he can do it himself only if he is doing what he calls "play." It takes a tremendous amount of skill to make therapy look casual. It may look like play to you, but actually both therapist and child are working very hard. All of the activities are purposeful; they are all directed toward a goal. And the goal is self-development or self-organization.

—Jean Ayres, 1979

Numerous therapeutic approaches are available for children with autism, including ABA, hippotherapy, nutritional therapy, craniosacral therapy, myofacial release, Floortime, and the list goes on. Some of these are considered controversial and some have been shown to be more helpful than others. Some alternative therapies have been reported to work very well in conjunction with use of a sensory based approach. Your child's OT may recommend trying some of these techniques. As a general rule, you should be very cautious with any new type of therapy approach and research it thoroughly before trying it with your child.

This chapter will detail some of the sensory-based strategies that may be used in an occupational therapy session in order to help improve your child's ability to tolerate or make sense of sensory input. Below is a breakdown of some of the most common treatment approaches. Please keep in mind that none of these therapeutic techniques should be attempted without the guidance of an accredited Occupational Therapist. Ultimately, however, your OT should be able to teach you—the parent—how to safely use many of these techniques with your child in your own home.

Treatment Approaches to Decrease Over-Responsivity

Brushing & Joint Compression

The Wilbarger Deep Pressure and Proprioceptive Technique (DPPT)

This technique was developed by Patricia Wilbarger, MEd, OTR, FAOTA, a clinical psychologist and an occupational therapist. For the past forty years, she has worked with children who have sensory processing disorders. Her method, based on implementing the use of

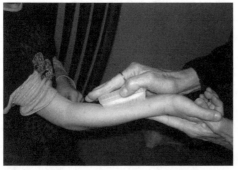
Figure 1

a soft surgical brush (see Figure 1) along with use of joint compression (see Figure 2), helps ready the brain to accept and organize information in a more acceptable and functional manner. Using a designated protocol, this technique provides stimulation that helps the brain improve its ability to organize sensory information specifically to the tactile, proprioceptive, and vestibular systems. The brushing program is used primarily for over-responsive children to help them achieve a relaxed, ready-to-learn state. Although

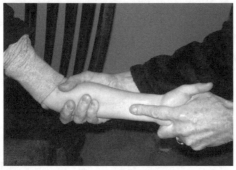
Figure 2

primarily used for kids with over-responsive systems, joint compression is also used to help organize kids with under-responsive systems. Some of the reported benefits of this technique include improved self-regulation or modulation of sensory input, ability to transition between activities, ability to attend or focus on an activity, and decreased tactile defensiveness.

Materials:
- Soft surgical brush, which is most effective in stimulating nerve endings in the skin.

Setting:
- OT room or clinic
- Home
- School

Method:
- Use the surgical brush to apply firm pressure to the surfaces of the child's hands, arms, back, legs, and feet. The brush is held in constant contact flat against the skin (or over the clothing). The brush travels up and down the body part slowly and without lifting. Avoid light pressure but do not press hard enough to cause pain or bruising.
- Joint compression should follow brushing. For this technique, the caregiver places his hands above and below the joint that is being compressed on the child, e.g., shoulders, elbows, wrists, fingers, hips, knees, ankles, and toes. For example, joint compression of the wrist involves one of the caregiver's hands on top of the child's hand and the caregiver's other hand above the child's wrist joint. (See Figure 2.) Both of the caregiver's hands push together towards the wrist, gently "squishing" the joint. Each joint is compressed ten consecutive times. Joint compression to the hips, knees, and feet can also be delivered by means of having the child jump up and down ten times.
- Initially brushing and joint compression should be performed every two hours for a number of days specified by your OT. This is because the input usually only lasts for ninety minutes and providing DPPT every two hours "re-

sets" the sensory system. Eventually, the amount of time can be reduced to specific times of distress for the child (e.g., transition times between classes or tasks, when child appears overwhelmed, etc.).

Precautions:
- Before attempting this technique, the caregiver should be thoroughly trained by an OT, who has completed a certified brushing program.
- It is essential that anyone being trained (teacher, aide, etc.) all use the same technique and degree of pressure.
- Never brush the child's stomach, chest, head, or neck.
- Only go back and forth, keeping the brush in constant contact with the skin.
- Never brush over a skin rash or sore.
- Always check the brush before using. It should be in good shape—not too soft or too scratchy.
- This technique should never cause physical pain or damage to the skin.

Many children will initially cry when this technique is being used. However, the majority begin to tolerate and actually enjoy this type of input. A downside of this technique is that it needs to be done at specific times (every two hours) and, more than likely, will not be carried out by the same person. Many parents report that their child responds better or worse depending on who is performing the technique because each person may provide the pressure in a slightly different manner.

Brushing with Textures
If the child does not tolerate DPPT and cries consistently during brushing, it is more than likely not being done correctly or efficiently. Another form of brushing, which appears to provide many of the same results listed above, as well as increasing awareness of tactile input to the hands, is to brush the child's hands with various textures using deep pressure (e.g., soft terry cloth washcloth, silky material, nylon body scrubber, etc.) instead of using a surgical brush. When this is first done, the therapist takes the child's hand and brushes with deep, firm pressure in one direction, then lifts the brush and starts back in the same spot. The child may respond by pulling his hand away. Dur-

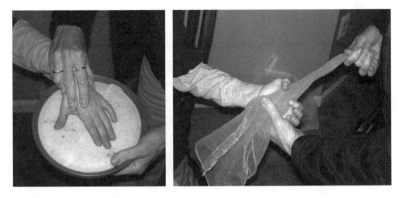

ing the next approach, the child is shown the object and the therapist gently holds the child's hand and asks if it can be done again. Usually, the child will allow this to happen and often will want more of this input. The purpose of brushing with textures is either to desensitize and increase tolerance for tactile input or help alert the child to textures with the long-term goal of increasing his participation in play and daily activities. Use of this technique not only appears to help the child to either calm or alert and organize but also provides the child the opportunity to accept or decline the input.

Materials:
- A variety of textured fabrics or objects, including soft, scratchy, Velcro, rubbery, plastic, etc.

Setting:
- A comfortable area in the home, e.g., a high chair, bean bag chair, etc., where the child will not wiggle around. The child can be sitting up or lying down as long as you have access to his hand.

Method:
- Test the texture on your own body first to be certain it is not painful or irritating.
- Use deep, firm pressure and always brush in same direction.
- While brushing the hands with various textures, use the opportunity to teach the names of the various textures, such as scratchy, soft, etc.

- As your child becomes more alert and tolerant of the brushing, you may want to place the textured objects in a box or bag and ask him to find the scratchy one, for example. This will also improve tactile discrimination, which will not begin until your child is more comfortable with tactile input.
- If there are specific items that your child seems to enjoy, provide him a small box of his preferred textures in an area of the home that he has access to and encourage him to brush his own hands with those objects throughout the day.

Precautions:

- Always monitor your child's response, looking to see if he alerts to the input or becomes upset with use of certain textures. If your child continues to show agitation with a specific texture, discontinue.
- Never brush over a skin rash or sore.
- This technique should never cause physical pain or damage to the skin.

Vestibular and Proprioceptive Input to Decrease Over-Responsivity

Vestibular and proprioceptive input can be used to alert or calm, depending on how it is needed. Below is a breakdown of some of the types of input that can be used to decrease an over-responsive

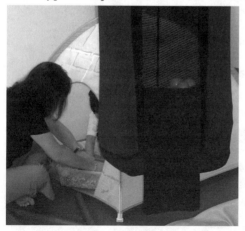

sensory system that registers small amounts of movement as "too much." The vestibular input used will be slow, gentle movement that will help calm and slowly desensitize the child's perception of movement in order to allow him to tolerate and learn from movement.

Materials:
- Platform swing
- Plastic bucket swing
- Blanket
- Hammock
- Wagon
- Rocking chair
- Ball pit

> *"The child is always in control of the amount of vestibular input received and is never pushed beyond his or her limits."* (Koomar & Bundy, 1991).

Setting:
- Calm, quiet area with minimal distractions
- Activities are simple and in view of your child so as not to surprise him

Methods:
- *Rocking* - Slow, gentle rocking only in one direction (i.e., back and forth *or* side to side) in a rocking chair or with the child on your lap on the floor
- *Deep pressure* -Your child may need to be snuggled into a hammock or wrapped in a blanket or tucked in a beanbag chair and then placed on a platform swing in order to tolerate the vestibular input (movement of the swing), at least at first
- *Singing or talking* to the child in a gentle, calm voice

Precautions:
- Always respect your child's fears—they are very real to him
- Avoid any sudden, fast, or jerky movements
- Monitor the child's reaction and only provide with the amount that he can tolerate

Tactile Activities to Decrease Over-Responsivity

Many children who are over-responsive to tactile input, especially to their hands, will avoid using their hands to play with or manipulate objects. Again, they perceive very small amounts of tactile input as painful. Any type of input to the hands needs to be introduced slowly and usually with deep, firm pressure. Below is a list of some of the activities that may be used to address tactile defensiveness to the hands.

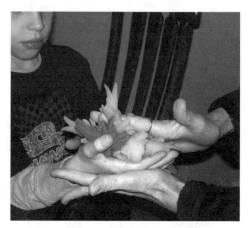

Materials:
- Vibrating toys or objects, playdough, pie or cookie dough, and various wet and dry textures

Setting:
- Sitting at a table in an OT room or clinic
- Sitting at a table at home
- Sitting at a table at school

Methods:
- *Vibration*—Introduce vibrating toys, such as plush toys with vibration, small plastic toys, Bumble Ball™. Initially, hand over hand deep pressure is applied. Your child's facial response is always monitored and objects are removed if he appears distressed. Slow, steady build-up of tolerance is used to increase acceptance and tolerance of the input.
- *Playdough*—Present playdough with hand over hand deep pressure and provide only to the level of tolerance that your child can handle. As your child slowly begins to tolerate the playdough, other activities can be introduced, such as rolling, pulling the dough apart, putting objects in and out of the dough. (You can also use edible playdough, cookie, or pie dough, especially if your child is likely to eat it).
- *Textures*—Brush hands with different textures (as listed above) and as your child slowly begins to tolerate certain types of textures, provide objects made of that texture in order to increase repertoire of objects. For example, if your child gravitates toward rubbery textures, give him soft squeeze toys of the same texture that provide cause/effect (e.g., sounds) or increase hand strength by squeezing.

❏ *Wet Textures*—Introduce shaving cream, whipped cream, lotions, etc. With deep pressure and hand over hand guidance, the therapist helps improve your child's tolerance for wet textures. Many children who are over-responsive may actually alert very well to these "strange" textures following initial input. As your child slowly begins to tolerate, activities could include making scribbles or shapes in the textures, moving hands in different directions (up, down, around and around). If your child refuses to touch wet textures, allow him to wear plastic gloves, paint with a paint brush, or touch liquid through a zip-top plastic bag. He will still experience the "feel" of these textures without actually touching them.

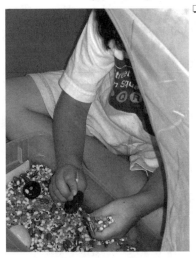

❏ *Dry Textures*—Use sand, rice, beans, etc. Textures are usually placed in a box or cafeteria type tray. To increase motivation, a favorite toy might be placed on top of the texture. Often your child will be motivated to pick up the toy and will slowly begin to tolerate the texture on his hand. As the tolerance increases, the toys can then be buried slightly under the texture, and eventually entirely buried in the texture.

Precautions:
- The therapist should proceed slowly and continually monitor your child's response, only upping the ante at the speed your child can handle it.
- The therapist should avoid surprising the child with a new toy or activity.

Treatment Activities to Improve an Under-Responsive Sensory System

Children who are under-responsive do not adequately register vestibular, tactile, or proprioceptive input and tend to crave large doses in their attempt to satisfy their sensory needs. Their high sensory thresholds require considerably more input before their brains register 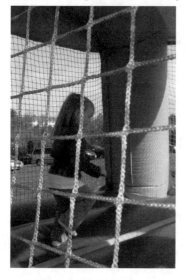 enough to respond to it. These kids can seem oblivious to their surroundings and not readily seek out sensory input, but more often than not they are described as always touching people or things, having difficulty knowing their boundaries or personal space, clumsy, unaware of their own strength, pressing too hard and breaking crayons or ripping the paper while they draw, throwing a ball too hard or with not enough force, and playing too rough with other children. Children with an under-responsive sensory system usually have a decreased ability to determine the amount of pressure needed to complete a task (e.g., to write on paper, throw a ball, or stack blocks). They often require very strong vestibular input and deep pressure activities. Deep pressure activities are used to help organize or alert their sensory systems.

Vestibular and Proprioceptive Input to Improve Under-Responsivity

Therapy sessions often focus on activities that help your child register sensory input more effectively. Following discussion with your child's OT, you can incorporate many of the following activities within the home.

Materials:
- Swings
- Trampolines

- Scooters
- Pads, mats, bolsters
- Tunnels
- Large therapy balls
- Climbing wall
- Tire tubes
- Ropes
- Trapeze
- Music

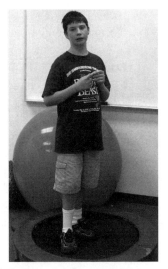

Setting:
- OT gym
- Large, open area at home

Methods:
- *Swings*—Playground swings and platform swings provide important input to the semi-circular canals in the ear, which are the major receptors for vestibular input. Try fast stop/start input, e.g., changing the direction of the swing from side to side, spinning, or back and forth. Use moving equipment to help improve balance and ability to remain on the swing while picking up an item on the floor or throwing a beanbag at a target, and later catching beanbags and trying to throw them on cards placed beneath them around the room.
- *Deep pressure or "heavy work"*—Engage the child in activities such as bouncing on a trampoline, tug of war, pushing objects, using their arms to pull himself around on a scooter board, jumping, and climbing.
- *Scooters*—Have your child lay on a scooter and roll down a small incline towards a designated target.
- *Obstacle courses*—Set up courses with activities to encourage moving the body through space and making the sensory system more aware of where the body is in relation to space. Encourage activities that promote moving the body over, under, in, out, up, down, and through various types of objects, like tunnels, bolsters, swings, and balance boards.
- *Rolling*—Have your child roll around on the floor and engage in activities such as rolling to a puzzle piece then rolling to

the other side of the room to connect it with other pieces.

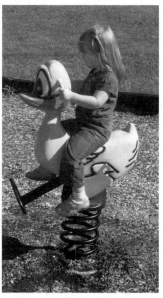

Precautions:
- Be aware of a change in voice, excessive giggling, flushed face, excessive talking, and dilated pupils, which may be signs of too much input.
- Vestibular input should only be provided by a trained therapist as vestibular input is a very powerful stimulus and too much may cause vomiting, heightened activity level, nausea, and drowsiness for up to eight hours following the input.
- Do not let your child spin excessively in one direction. After three or four rotations, stop the swing and start spinning in the opposite direction.

Tactile Activities to Increase Tactile Discrimination

A variety of activities will be used to help your child learn how to differentiate information from an object he receives through touch, and improve the amount of pressure needed to manipulate specific objects (e.g., pencil, blocks, ball, etc.). Below is a list of activities that might be used to achieve this goal.

Materials:
- Playdough
- Squeeze/stress balls
- Rubber toys that light up or make sounds
- Plastic accordion tubes
- Soft textures items (silk scarves, stuffed animals)
- Beads
- Velcro
- Vibrating toys
- Tub of sand, rice, or beans

Setting:
- OT room or clinic
- Home
- School

Methods:
- *Vibration*—The use of vibrating objects may help your child become more aware of input to his hands. One type of activity could be use of a vibrating pen to increase your child's ability to hold onto the pen while he is making shapes, writing his name, etc. A vibrating Bumble Ball™ may alert your child and increase his motivation to turn it off and on.
- *Playdough*—The use of playdough provides deep pressure. Activities such as pressing cookie cutters into the dough, and burying objects and pulling them out with fingers will not only help improve tactile awareness but will strengthen the muscles of the hands. Use of cookie dough can also provide heavy work and can be used to perform a functional task, such as making cookies, which requires following directions.

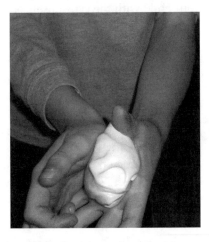

- *Brushing hands*—Brushing with different textures helps "wake up" the hands. It also helps your child begin to tolerate different textures and learn how to discriminate (identify) different textures. Ask your child to list different attributes of a texture (e.g., a wooden block is hard, square, small) with him looking at the object as you brush his hand with it. Later, place the object in a small bag and have your child identify the item by touch. Initially, you may want to have two of the same object (one hidden in the bag and another out in plain view). As his discrimination skills improve, eliminate the visible one.

■ *Heavy work activities*—These activities will not only provide tactile input to the hands but will also provide important input to the muscles and joints of the arms and legs. Try household chores such as ripping up junk mail, stacking cans or books on a shelf, using a squirt bottle to water plants or clean a window, wiping off a table.

We've just discussed a small sampling of the techniques that are commonly used with children who demonstrate a sensory processing disorder. These same principles are used regardless of the child's primary diagnosis, whether it is AD/HD, LD, or autism. Often, children with autism will display behaviors that could be motivated by either a sensory processing problem or autism. An experienced therapist will be able to begin to tease out which behaviors are due to what and provide your child with the type of sensory input that will help him improve his ability to tolerate sensory input. The main idea is to provide your child with the "just right" amount of input (for him) in order to begin to "make sense" of sensory information. Your OT will regularly change up the activities that your child does in therapy—upping the ante when he shows signs that he is ready. For example, while your child lays on a platform swing, the OT may throw beanbags for him to catch. Later, he'll be asked to drop the beanbags on different colored paper on the floor as he swings about the room. In this way, she is increasing the demands made on his sensory system with the goal of improving his ability to process input.

A Sample Treatment Session

Morgan

Morgan is the now four-year-old child with autism who we first met in Chapter 2. He has been going to weekly private OT sessions for the past year, mainly to address issues related to poor sensory processing. He experiences tactile defensiveness to his hands and feet, fear of movement, and poor body awareness. Morgan provides no eye contact and seems happiest just laying on the floor and talking to his hands. (He holds his hands in front of his face and moves them similar to a puppet.) His mother's goals for therapy include increasing

Morgan's ability to hold objects, such as a spoon or marker, teaching him to help with dressing, and increasing his ability to play with toys more appropriately.

Since therapy has begun, Morgan has made slow, steady progress. An important factor in Morgan's success is the ongoing carryover of techniques from therapy to home. Through slow, gentle input (at a pace agreeable to him) he can now tolerate being on a swing and will often lay on his belly and push the swing back and forth with his feet. He also enjoys going up and down a small slide. At home, Morgan now likes to play on his swing set and enjoys running around the yard, chasing the dog. He is now able to hold a marker and is beginning to color small, simple objects. Morgan has improved his ability to brush his teeth and can scoop and feed himself ice cream without constant reminders not to use his hands. These achievements have not come easy but are a result of weekly therapy sessions, which have not only provided the right amount of sensory input, but continue to provide him time and confidence to find the "just right" level of challenge to engage in an activity. With each session, his family is improving not only their skills but their ability to "tease out" what is sensory-related and what is an autistic-like behavior.

A typical therapy session for Morgan goes something like this: Morgan enters the room, which has been slightly darkened in order to decrease excessive visual stimuli. A picture schedule of activities that will be addressed during this session is on the wall and reviewed with Morgan. He takes off his shoes and is seated in a small, snug chair that provides some deep pressure. The session begins with a greeting song during which Morgan needs constant reminders to sit and engage. He continues to get out of the chair and begins to push his head and body into the therapist. The therapist provides deep pressure to his arms and shoulders and sits him back in the chair. Morgan is provided hand-over-hand help with removing the "greeting" card from the picture schedule posted on the wall.

Next, the OT brushes Morgan with a surgical brush and provides him with joint compression. She sings a "brushing song" as Morgan looks at her, smiles, and sings along. (Brushing and joint compression have alerted Morgan's system to begin to work.) With cues, he removes the activity schedule's "brushing" card and replaces it with the "play" card. At this time, Morgan is offered two choices: trampoline or box of toys. He chooses a box of toys, which contains many types of fidgets, including rubber balls, stretchy frogs, stress balls, resistive tubes, Koosh balls, and a flashlight. His therapist provides him with a small bolster pillow to sit on while playing with the objects. The bolster provides proprioceptive and vestibular input as he slowly rocks on it from side to side.

Although initially Morgan refused to hold objects, the fidget toys have helped him to slowly begin to tolerate tactile input. The textures of the fidget toys are all different but the resistive, rubbery

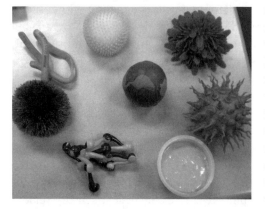

components are providing some heavy work to his hands and this helps calm and organize his sensory system. Inspecting each fidget object visually alerts him. Although there are some fidgets that Morgan tends to self-stim with (only wants to play with the toy in one rigid way) the therapist has been able to increase Morgan's repertoire of activities by slowly substituting other objects that provide sensory input but decrease the stimming.

To encourage imitation, the OT will engage in parallel play with Morgan, or simultaneously perform the same action as Morgan. Once he's engaged, they can take turns initiating actions. The OT picks up a rubber ball with a loop attached and threads her finger in the loop. Morgan watches and when the therapist hands him the toy, he also tries to thread his finger, allowing the OT to help him. Morgan bounces the ball and on two occasions he looks up at the therapist and smiles at his achievement. The therapist notices that Morgan is grinding his teeth so she provides him with a chewy tube (small rubber tube). Morgan eagerly takes the tube and places it in his mouth as he continues to explore the toys. The tube is providing some heavy work to his mouth and helping him to continue to focus on play.

After five more minutes of fine motor play the therapist initiates a clean up song and Morgan helps the therapist pick up the toys. Morgan then picks the next card on the activity chart, the ball pit. Morgan loves to fully immerse his body in the balls and begins to "talk" to his hands. The therapist gets in the ball pit with him and scoops up some of the plastic balls in a laundry basket. She lifts the basket and says, "Ready...set..." Morgan looks up and says, "Go!" He watches the balls drop and smiles. The therapist then places the basket over Morgan's head and asks where he is. After a minute, he lifts the basket from his head and smiles at the therapist. While the balls are providing Morgan with deep pressure, the therapist's goal at this time is to try to engage Morgan in interactive play. Next, the OT initiates dancing. This activity provides deep pressure and vestibular input (alerting) as Morgan swings around and drops down into the balls. After five minutes the therapist sings a song signaling that the activity is over. Morgan begins to whine and pushes himself further down into the balls. As the therapist continues to sing, she also counts to three. This consistent structure and routine seems to help Morgan comply with the request to get out of the ball pit. Although still whining, he exits the ball pit and is moved to another area of the room where his activity chart is.

The next activity card is a picture of a desk. Morgan, familiar with the routine, goes and sits on a therapy ball at the desk. The OT gives Morgan the chewy tube again as sitting activities are very difficult for him and the chewing resistance seems to help him calm, organize, and focus. On the desk is a chart with three pictures of activities that will be done while seated. One activity involves placing stickered clothespins onto the side of containers matching stickers. This task not only helps with fine motor skills (strength and eye-hand coordination) but is resistive and considered heavy work (to squeeze the clothespins open). He completes the task without any help and sets out to complete the next task, which is coloring. Morgan is not as excited about this task and the therapist needs to redirect him twice. She places her hands on his shoulders and sings a song as she bounces him up and down on the ball. This provides deep pressure and helps to alert Morgan's system to follow directions and engage in the task. Following the input, Morgan is able to finish the coloring task independently. The last activity acts mostly as a reward. Morgan grabs the large container filled with macaroni noodles, and although there are items in the box to scoop and pour, he opts to place his hands and arms into the noodles and wiggle them around. This not only provides tactile input but deep pressure to Morgan's arms. He reacts by smiling and softly singing a song. The session ends with Morgan returning to a chair to put on his shoes and socks.

When Morgan first began therapy he did not seem to be aware of his feet, and for many of the early sessions, his therapist would provide lots of deep pressure and tactile input to his feet before putting on his shoes. Morgan is now not only more aware of his feet but can put on shoes and socks, requiring help only to tie them. His mother is pleased that Morgan is now beginning to help with dressing and they are working on buttoning buttons and tying shoes.

Finally, Morgan takes the last card off the activity chart. He and his OT sing a goodbye song while the therapist provides deep pressure to Morgan's hands and arms. Good eye contact is noted when he is asked to say good-bye. As Morgan quietly plays with a toy in the waiting room, the last five minutes of the session are devoted to reviewing many of the activities and strategies used during the session so Morgan's mother can carry them over to the home environment.

Can a Parent Use This Type of Therapy At Home?

Often, parents are under the impression that their child only benefits from the activities during the one hour therapy sessions. However, for therapy to work, it is imperative that the child use the sensory strategies within his familiar everyday routine. Your child's OT will discuss with you how she conducts treatment and her rationale should be fully explained. Following a treatment session, the OT should provide recommendations on how to set up your home environment, such as establishing a "chill out" area or an area for more input. She'll also describe how to carry out activities that your child enjoyed or tolerated during the OT session.

Therapy at home should be introduced as play, using some of the techniques that your child seemed to either enjoy or alert to during the therapy session. For example, using squishy balls or playdough to provide deep pressure, brushing the hands with various types of textures, or providing times for your child to use a swing or bounce on a ball. In order to work, therapy at home should be enjoyable and fit into your family's routine. Your child's sensory issues should improve through the daily carryover of input. You and your child will feel empowered as you begin to determine what works and what doesn't. The following chapter, Your Child's Sensory Diet, will provide information about how to incorporate therapy into your daily routine.

9 Your Child's Sensory Diet

A sensory diet can be incorporated into all aspects of daily life and within any setting. A sensory diet plan is ideal as a structure for home programs that treat sensory processing problems. It is also a powerful adjunct to school, work or early intervention.
—Wilbarger, 1995

In previous chapters we discussed how children with sensory processing disorder benefit from regularly scheduled therapy services with a trained OT. Activities addressed within the sessions are individualized and intended to improve your child's specific sensory processing issues. However, sessions are usually only once a week and last about an hour. What can you do to continue to help your child when he's not in therapy? What is your family to do on a daily basis when your child continues to struggle with his ability to process sensory information in an effective way? This chapter will provide information about sensory diets and how to use one with your child at home and in the community. It will provide ideas for environmental adaptations, therapeutic strategies that can be integrated into your child's daily routine (i.e., during dressing, feeding, playing), along with and suggestions for putting your child more at ease in various settings during stressful situations or when there has been a shift in routine. The ideas are broken down into sections for calming, alerting, and organizing activities to help your child regulate his sensory system and be ready to engage and participate in play and daily tasks.

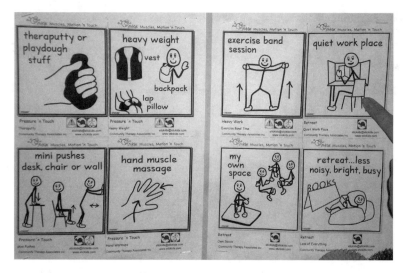

The term "sensory diet" was coined by Wilbarger and Wilbarger (1991). The concept was developed to explain sensory processing more concisely to families of children with a sensory processing disorder. *A sensory diet is a specific and individualized combination of sensory activities provided throughout the day that enables a person's sensory system to either calm or alert and allow adequate sensory input for an optimal state of arousal.* This optimal state—at once calm *and* alert—is necessary in order for your child to learn and attend to new learning experiences in compliance with the demands of the environment. Use of a sensory diet enables a child with sensory processing issues to take in information at a pace that works for his particular sensory system. Just as food nourishes our bodies, a sensory diet helps to nourish our brains with pertinent sensory information. Using a sensory diet will provide either a "meal" (long-lasting input, such as deep pressure) or a "snack" (short-term input that one might get from squeezing a stress ball). A sensory diet provides structure and a concrete way for families to help their children learn how to regulate their sensory system. It has become a common practice to use a sensory diet for children with autism and many occupational therapists recommend its use for home and school.

Your child's sensory diet is initiated by the OT during his initial evaluation, when various types of sensory input are provided and tested out. These might include brushing, deep pressure activities, observing your child's response to swings, trampolines, or small objects such as squishy balls and playdough. Depending on your child's response to this input, activities will be recommended to try throughout the day at home. Information gleaned from parent reporting, for example, "My child does not hold objects and is constantly moving," along with information about times of the day that your child is either overly alert or seems lethargic, will also be taken into account. The results of a Sensory Profile—a detailed sensory questionnaire filled out by a family member (see Chapter 4)—will also provide valuable information for setting up the sensory diet. The profile breaks down various areas of sensory functioning and can determine if your child is primarily a "sensory-seeker" or "sensory-avoider" or displays a combination of both throughout his day.

There is no cookbook approach to developing a sensory diet in that every child's sensory needs will be different. The sensory diet is a dynamic program—it will constantly be revised and updated both through therapeutic intervention and use of various activities that you and your child's therapist feel may be working. Once a daily sensory diet is begun, families are encouraged to keep a diary for a few days, including times of the day when behaviors seem out of control or the child tends to lay on floor with limited participation in any activity. The diary should also include the child's positive or negative response to the recommended sensory strategies. The ultimate purpose of the sensory diet is to help your child achieve that calm/alert state or, to use another term, self-regulation—being in the "just right" state to begin to understand and use sensory information effectively in order for learning to happen.

As stated throughout this book, every child is different and will need a specific sensory diet. Below is a list of simple guidelines to follow when using a sensory diet:

- DO *develop a daily routine*. Start out simple and determine times when using sensory strategies will work best, e.g., upon waking, after meals, after school, before bedtime.
- DO *determine activities or objects that are motivating to your child*. This may help to increase compliance, especially for children who need calming.
- DO *choose appropriate activities* according to your child's age, level of awareness, and ability to engage and tolerate the sensory input. The sensory activities should be pleasant and feel good to your child.
- DO *try novel approaches* and allow yourself to think outside the box. If your child won't hold a pencil but loves playdough, wrap a clump of playdough around a pencil

and have him grasp it there. If your child has a fascination with cars, incorporate toy cars into sensory activities.

- DO *add variety.* For the child who needs alerting, varying activities is a good idea. You may need to move slowly for the child who needs calming activities but gradually increase his repertoire of sensory activities so he doesn't learn to only tolerate certain things.

- DO *watch your child's response to input.* If his face is relaxed or he is attending, this is a good sign. If he is crying, screaming, or laughing too hard it is most likely his way of saying it's too much. If your child is a "sensory avoider," move slowly but be consistent.

- DO *continue to consult with your child's OT* for new ideas or when it may be time to up the ante or begin to incorporate some functional activities into the diet (e.g., dressing, using a pencil, etc.).

- DO *try to use the sensory input and incorporate into a functional task* (e.g., provide deep pressure by kneading cookie dough; provide vibration by using a mixer to help make dinner).

- DO *try to tease out which behaviors are related to the diagnosis of autism* (if the child is on the spectrum) *versus which are related to sensory processing challenges.* How you address these behaviors will depend on the reasons behind them.

- DO *remember that sensory input may not always work the same way every day.* Your child will have good and bad days and this will often depend on variables out of your control, e.g., the child did not sleep well the night before.

- DON'T *force activities* when your child is truly upset or "bouncing off the walls."

- DON'T *hang your hopes on the sensory diet working immediately or "curing" your child of autism.* It's a slow, consistent process and your child needs time to feel comfortable.

Keep in mind that the following sensory activities are only suggestions and may or may not work for your child. It is highly recommended that you have your child work closely with an OT who is experienced in treating children with SPD, as she will be able to guide both you and your child through this ever-evolving process.

Achieving the Optimal State of Arousal

Children with autism often engage in perseverative or obsessive-type behaviors. This may be linked to their diagnosis of autism but may also be the result of a poor sensory processing system. For example, spinning oneself or objects (self-stimulation) may be a sensory seeker's way of getting visual and vestibular input. A sensory avoider might resist change and like things to stay the same in an effort to limit his amount of sensory input. In fact, the majority of children with sensory issues will display both over- *and* under-responsive reactions. As you will learn from working with your OT, your child may fluctuate between experiencing an over- and under-responsive sensory system (for example, under-responsive to proprioceptive input but overly sensitive to auditory input). For this reason, a sensory diet includes a combination of alerting, organizing, or calming activities (Kranowitz, 1998).

Throughout the day, your child's sensory system may need varying "doses" of either alerting or calming input, depending upon the circumstances, environment, and the behaviors that he is displaying. The child who is under-responsive will benefit from alerting or organizing activities. The child who is over-responsive is easily over-stimulated and will often display either a "fight or flight" response or "shut-down." This child will respond best to calming activities that provide slow, steady input and help the sensory system modulate and calm. Although it may sound confusing, "heavy work" will benefit either an over- or under-responsive sensory system by providing the just right input for the child to modulate. To illustrate, the deep pressure provided by pulling a wagon filled with books will calm an over-responsive child, whereas the same activity will alert the brain of an under-responsive child by contracting his muscles.

Alerting

Alerting techniques are used if your child appears to be under-responsive to sensory input. This child may not respond to his environment or the people around him or he might respond in the opposite fashion, running and crashing into walls and furniture, always touching people or objects, constantly mouthing objects, and spinning without getting dizzy. He might also be a messy eater or have decreased fine motor or sequencing skills needed for dressing or playing with toys. If your child has some of these behaviors, he is described as a *sensory seeker*—constantly seeking out sensory input that will "wake up," or alert his system. This is his effort to try to modulate or organize his sensory system but usually meets with limited success.

If your child is under-responsive to sensory input his OT might recommend that you set up an area in your home devoted to alerting his senses. Provide toys and activities here that will give him opportunities to obtain vestibular and proprioceptive input. Decorate this environment with visually alerting colors and bright lights (i.e., fluorescent bulbs, disco lights, a small flashing traffic light). Provide auditorially stimulating music and consider incorporating a scent known to be alerting, such as peppermint, wintergreen, grapefruit, or lemon.

Alerting Proprioceptive Activities

Proprioception is our awareness of where our body is in relation to space. Proprioceptive activities, especially "heavy work," provide deep pressure to our joints and muscles, which, in this case, will be calming to the brain. This feedback can be especially beneficial before under-responsive kids are expected to sit down and do a task that requires concentration, like homework or playing a board game. It's a good idea to provide brief action/movement breaks such as jumping jacks, hopping on one foot, or a relay race from one end of room to the other. Other ideas to incorporate into your child's day include:

- Resistive-type work, such as vacuuming, lifting a bag of newspapers, taking out recyclables, wiping off a chalkboard or kitchen table
- Pushing or pulling, e.g., a wagon or cart filled with objects
- Hitting and catching a bean-filled ball
- Batting a balloon or a balloon on a tether
- Physical activities like push-ups, wheel barrel walks, army crawl, animal walks (e.g., crab, bear)
- Crashing into large pillows or a beanbag chair
- Playground activities such as hanging from monkey bars or using a climbing wall
- Playing movement games such as 'Follow the Leader,' 'Red Light/Green Light,' or 'Red Rover'
- Pushing or walking a ball up a wall

- Setting up and navigating through an obstacle course that allows lots of body movement (jumping over a box, squeezing under a chair, crawling through a tunnel, etc.)
- Doing simple yoga or Pilates positions
- Jumping on a trampoline
- Dancing to music, e.g., Hip Hop or the 'Hokey Pokey'
- Pulling up on a rope or chin bar
- Pushing big toy trucks in sand or dirt
- Supervised wrestling or roughhousing
- Playing basketball with a Nerf™ ball
- Doing push-ups with hands against a wall
- Crawling around the room to locate items in a scavenger hunt
- Jumping games such as hopscotch and jumping rope
- Bouncing a ball to a rhyme or interactive song
- Lying on a scooter board and pushing with hands to different areas of the room
- Playing 'Tug of War'
- Games such as London Bridges, Simon Says, charades (using large movements that require motor planning)

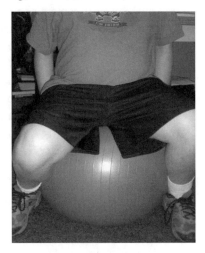

- Writing letters with your finger on child's back
- Lying over a therapy ball and reading a book or walking on hands to do a puzzle
- Doing wall or chair push ups
- Relay races
- Running around in a safe area in the home
- Marching games, dancing, hopping, spinning
- Jumping activities such as jumping off a low bench into a pile of pillows
- Interactive video games, such as Wii™ System

Alerting Vestibular Activities

Like proprioception, the vestibular system gathers information through movement, but more in response to how our movements are affected by gravity. The receptors for vestibular input are located in the inner ear, which sense movement of the head, and are, in part, responsible for balance. The following activities are stimulating and alerting to the vestibular system:

- Fast, unpredictable movements on a swing, e.g., rotary spinning, stop/start, changing the direction of the swing
- Sitting, bouncing, or rolling on a therapy ball or wiggle cushion (inflatable disc cushion)
- Playground activities such as swings, sliding board
- Using a Sit 'n' Spin toy (monitor that the child does not do to excess)
- 'Body bowling' wherein your child lays flat on the ground with legs and arms tight to the body and rolls his body to knock down plastic or spongy bowling pins or targets
- Games such as 'Ring Around the Rosie,' 'Here We Go 'Round the Mulberry Bush'
- Playing tag or running from one side of the room to the other
- Somersaults
- Balancing on a balance beam
- Dancing
- Pretending to be an airplane and "flying" to a different area of the room
- Doing exercises that involve moving the head in different directions

Keep in mind that you can incorporate a learning component into many of these activities. Often you will see the child want to continue to engage in a certain sensory activity (e.g., swinging, bouncing on a ball, playing with playdough) and you'll know that he is alerting to the input. Once you see this, it's your opportunity to place more demands on him to listen and learn new skills. For example, ask him to hop three times, or spin to the right three times, then left three times, or run to the red chair to pick up a toy then skip over and place it on the blue desk. Likewise, you can engage your child in deskwork, a board game, or a puzzle while they're sitting and bouncing on a large therapy ball.

Sensory-seekers will often seek out large amounts of vestibular (e.g., excessive spinning) or proprioceptive (e.g., constant crashing) feedback without ever calming down. If this is noted, impose structure on the activity by means of adding a cognitive conmponent. For example, ask the child to spin three times to the right and then answer a question, spell a word, etc. before spinning to the left three times. Engaging their minds in this way will help them register the sensory input more effectively.

Alerting Tactile Activities

Just under the skin are receptors that gather information through touch. This is our tactile sensory system. Activities that alert our tactile system include:

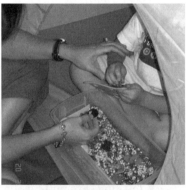

- Tickling
- Vibration (use toys, toothbrushes, and pens that vibrate)
- Squeezing or pulling odd textures such as Koosh™ balls, rubbery or stretchy toys, loofas, Velcro, squeeze balls or toys
- Brushing child's hands with odd textures (e.g., rubbery, scratchy, silky) in order to alert or "wake up" the hands

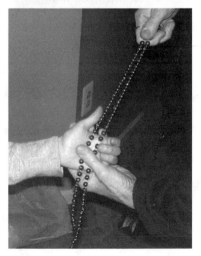

- Pressing Mardi Gras beads against child's palm and running beads through the hand with deep pressure
- Vigorous rubbing with towel to body and hair following bathing
- Playing with textures such as sand, rice, or playdough (bury small

preferred toys in the material and have the child find the toy and brush off all of the texture with his fingers)

- Rolling playdough out into long strips and making letters using templates

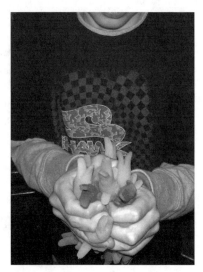

- Allowing child to stick their hand into a "feely bag" (a bag filled with sensory toys or textures listed above)

- Popping and squeezing bubble wrap

- Touching or "drawing" with shaving cream, finger paints, Jell-o, gel, pudding

- Using manipulatives to build towers

- Pressing Wikki Stix™ (plastic coated, bendable strings) into letter shapes or patterns

- Using squirt bottles to water plants

- Pulling Velcro balls off a Velcro target

- Cutting out items of heavy poster board or foam

- Pushing in or pulling out foam puzzle pieces

- Water play, e.g., squeezing sponges, filling water bottles using a turkey baster (in a tub, sink, or bucket)

- Putting stickers on fingertips

- Use of fidgets to hold during lesson time

- Clapping or finger play games, e.g., 'Where is Thumbkin?'

Alerting Auditory Activities

Sounds can be soothing or stimulating. To alert your child's auditory system try the following:

- Alter the volume and pitch of your voice to increase your child's attention to sound

- Make up songs or rhymes for various daily activities, e.g., a bathing sequence, "This is the way we wash your arm,

up and down, up and down," while you have your child
help with the task

- Record different sounds and then ask your child to match
the sound with the object that makes that sound
- Play rhyming games or tap out a rhythm on the table where
the child fills in the rhyming word or imitates the taps
- Use a ticking timer or novelty talking clock to alert the
child to specific activities

Alerting Visual Activities

We all know from our own experience that objects that are bright
and colorful capture our attention better than those of neutral tones.
Incorporate color into visual activities to alert your child, such as:

- Playing games such as Simon where different colors light
up and the child must reproduce the pattern
- Color with highlighter pens
- Play 'Eye Spy' by shining a flashlight on various items in a
darkened room
- Hide familiar or preferred toys in textures or a box and
have your child find them

Alerting Oral Motor Activities

We feel *and* taste things with our mouth, so oral motor activities
provide a double whammy in alerting our sensory systems. Our sense of
smell also plays a hand in our sense of taste. Have your child who is under-responsive try some of these techniques to "wake up" his mouth:

- Taste test strange or interesting flavors, e.g., spicy foods,
sour candies or flavored candy sprays, pickles, tart foods,
such as lemons, to "wake-up" the mouth
- Suck on cold items like ice, popsicles, or frozen fruit
- Chew crunchy foods such as chips, raw veggies, crackers, pretzels, or resistive foods such as licorice, gummy
worms, or fruit roll ups
- Play with mouth toys or instruments that vibrate or make
your lips vibrate, e.g., vibrating toothbrushes, kazoos, harmonicas, Jews' harps, trumpets, saxophones, harmonicas
- Chew flavored gum, gummy worms

- Drink beverages with strong, sour, or citrus flavors, e.g., cranberry or lemonade
- Apply flavored lip gloss with strong scents
- Smear a small amount of chocolate or peanut butter on different areas of your child's lips and have him locate it with his tongue and lick it off
- Use straws to blow cotton balls or packing peanuts towards a target
- Blow through a straw into shaving cream or paint to create a picture
- Use whistles that produce a sound or cause an action
- Blow pinwheels or bubbles
- Lick lollipops that rotate on a base when activated

Alerting Olfactory Activities

Certain scents—such as peppermint, wintergreen, grapefruit, basil, tangerine, and lemon—are noted to be alerting and help improve concentration. Incorporate these into activities to alert your child who is under-responsive.

- Put a small drop of a strong scent, e.g., perfume, on a cotton ball and allow your child to smell it
- Apply a small amount of cleaning product with a strong scent to a sponge and allow them to help with clean-up
- Have your child sniff various scents and have him match up the scents with pictures of the objects that smell that way (e.g., peppermint with candy cane)

Children who are sensory-seekers should be provided alerting stimulation throughout the day, but keep in mind that these kids can also become over-stimulated and may need time to calm down or regroup. Although we mainly think of using calming activities with children who are over-repsonsive to too much stimulation, be aware that children who are under-repsonsive may become "over wound" and begin to act very silly. Winding down in a "chill out" space may be necessary. (See the next section for information on calming techniques.)

Calming

Calming techniques are used if your child is *over-responsive* to sensory input. A child who is over-responsive is overly aware of his environment and appears to be anxious and nervous in response to everyday input and will often exhibit behaviors such as increased crying or irritation with noise, movement, or touching objects. More than likely, this child does not like new activities, using his hands, having people too close to him, and may be particular about clothing and food textures. This child is described as a *sensory avoider*—he avoids many types of sensory input (i.e., tactile, vestibular, oral, auditory) and perceives such input as noxious or dangerous. As a result, he may exhibit a "fight or flight" response and more than likely miss out on opportunities to explore and learn from sensory input unless he engages in activities that help to modulate his sensory systems. Once he is in a calm state, he will feel safer and should have an increased tolerance for sensory input.

Environment can have a major impact on whether your child is able to calm, alert, or organize his sensory system to all types of sensory input he experiences in his environment. If your child is over-responsive to his environment, his reaction may be either to withdraw or scream in response to input. You may notice that your child is over-stimulated after a full day of school, a trip to the mall, a birthday party, or just a noisy meal. The constant bombardment of all types of sensations and his attempts to make sense of them can be exhausting and may have a cumulative effect. If we try to imagine how we feel when we have had that type of day, most would agree that we just want some quiet time with no interruptions. Your child will need help learning how to decrease over-stimulation to his senses and find a calm state.

One way to do this is to provide a "chill-out area," or a quiet area in your home where your child can go to decompress and regroup. The area should be a place that is quiet and free from too much sensory stimulation (noise, lights, etc.). When your child seems overwhelmed, take him to this area so he learns to identify it as a place that will help him relax and feel comfortable. A chill-out area can be created fairly inexpensively using objects you already have around your home. Try to incorporate the following features:

- Choose a darkened or dimly lit, quiet area of the home (avoid rooms with fluorescent lighting)

- Keep the area simple and free of visual distractions and clutter (not too many bright colors or objects)
- Provide a small tent, create a fort by draping blankets over a table, or convert a small closet or a large cardboard box into a safe space
- Rooms with carpets will likely be less aversive than tile or hardwood floor
- Blankets and pillows for the child to wrap up in
- Bean bag or rocking chair
- Soft calming music with slow, even beat or preferred music (with headphones if tolerated)
- Familiar books or storybook tapes
- Kaleidoscopes and gel filled wands with sparkles
- Soft or novel lights such as a Lava lamp, twinkling lights, or night light (avoid rapidly flickering lights)
- Fish tank or aquarium
- Bag of favorite toys (i.e., Beanie Babies, soft squeeze toys, rubbery objects)
- Visual charts of the day's activities to help prepare your child for changes in his routine. Use a watch or timer (visual timers without sound work well) to help smooth transitions
- Provide a chair that allows your child's feet to be in contact with the floor (helps him feel grounded)

If possible, avoid providing your child with his favorite stimming object in the chill-out area so he won't just "zone out." Instead encourage him to use some of the other items listed above. (This is usually easier said than done.) If you must, initially let your child have his favorite stimming object but begin to substitute other items that he shows an interest in. Encourage him to play with these items and slowly fade out the stimming toys from the chill-out area. Following are some other recommendations that may help to calm your child's sensory system.

Calming Proprioceptive Activities
- Vibrating pillows or toys (monitor for tolerance)
- Deep pressure rubs, e.g., back, head
- Rubbing lotion on arms, legs, back, etc.

- Being snuggled up in a beanbag chair or wrapped in blankets; covering body (not head) with a heavy quilt or under a weighted blanket
- Wrapping arms or legs with ace bandages (not too tight)
- Brushing the skin with a therapy brush and using joint compression (see Chapter 8)
- 'Hot Dog Game' wherein child is wrapped in a blanket or sleeping bag and deep pressure is provided to his back while you sing a simple rhythmic song
- Wedging beanbags around your child's body (possibly at bedtime)
- Providing deep pressure to child's hips as he gently bounces on a ball (child's feet planted on the floor for balance)
- Digging in dirt or sand with a shovel
- Wearing a heavy backpack (filled with books, toys, or canned food) or a weighted vest, or lap or neck pad weighted down with beans, rice, or sand
- Snuggling child in a beanbag chair and slowly rocking side to side to a rhythmic song

Calming Vestibular Activities *(often work hand in hand with proprioceptive input)*

- Gentle linear (back/forth) movement like from a swing or rocking chair. (Note: Movements should always be predictable and rhythmic. If child feels vulnerable in an open swing, try a bucket swing that has sides and a front. If not feasible, sit on the swing and have the child sit on your lap providing a snug space.)
- Jumping or marching in place (possibly placing your hands on your child's hips, providing deep pressure) to rhythmic songs or chants
- Wrapping in a blanket (without breathing or vision blocked) and slowly rolling on the floor from one spot to the next

Calming Tactile Activities

- Deep pressure activities (e.g., being snuggly wrapped in a warm blanket)

- Deep pressure to the hands
  - "Sandwich" activities, such as lying under weighted items, e.g., heavy quilt, or pillow filled with beans, sand, or rice
- Back rubs (deep pressure with constant skin to skin contact)
- Tight or snug fitting clothing, such as those made with spandex or Lycra (i.e., Danskin™, Under-Armour™, or Nike™). (Note: These can be worn under regular clothing.)
- Use of a weighted vest (commercial) or a vest with pockets and small weights placed inside them, lap blanket, belt, or weighted neck pillow
- Putting lotion on arms and legs with firm deep pressure
- Vigorous rubbing with towel to body and hair following bathing
- Squeezing a zip-type bag filled with products such as styling gel, shaving cream, finger paints, which allows your child to experience them without actually having to touch them
- Brushing program (see more about this in Chapter 10)
- Soaking in warm water
- Slowly introducing different textures (e.g., if he tolerates sand, you can have him make shapes and letters in the sand with his fingers versus using a pencil)
- Allow the child to wear gloves to increase his tolerance for aversive textures
- Playing in a ball pit

Note: Avoid light or unexpected touch and always approach your child from the front where he can see you and what you are doing.

Calming Auditory Activities

Noise can be a particularly challenging form of sensory input for children with ASD and SPD. They often perceive even everyday common noises as painful. Make your best effort to empathize with your child's responses to noise. Avoid using a loud voice; try to talk with a calm, firm voice with an even tempo, even if your child has done something that made you angry. When possible, prepare your child for a loud or unexpected noise, e.g., before you turn on the blender or garbage disposal. When in public, steer your child away from noisy areas like food courts or chatty people. Monitor your child's behavior in crowded or loud places and, if possible, find a place where you can take him to help calm or decrease the extra auditory input. Consider providing your child with soft ear plugs or fabric headbands that may help muffle or dampen sounds. If your child seems upset with sounds that you cannot identify, look around the room carefully, as some children cannot even tolerate the gentle clicking sound of a wall clock or the hum of a fluorescent light. (Conversely, some children may respond well to those kinds of background noises and will calm to the sound of a fan, vacuum, or bubbling aquarium.) Your child may actually show more tolerance to sounds if he is the one in control of, say, flushing the toilet, or turning the volume up on a radio. Some children may increase their tolerance to sound using the strategy of counting to five before turning on the vacuum cleaner or blender. In addition to these suggestions, try increasing your child's tolerance for auditory stimulation using the following activities:

- Tape record various everyday sounds and make pictures of the objects making the sound (telephone, ambulance, etc.). Make a game of finding the picture to go along with the sound.
- Provide deep pressure and hugs to help your child calm when he is upset by sounds.
- Try to encourage your child to tolerate and listen to music through headphones, especially when in a new or noisy environment.

Calming Visual Activities

Visual stimulation can also be a big trigger for kids with ASD and SPD. When your child is experiencing stress, if possible take him to his chill-out space. If that's not possible, dim the lights. Have your child wear sunglasses, a large brim hat, or sun visor (if tolerated) when in a bright or sunny area. Do not demand that your child always look at your face as this may be very overwhelming to his visual system. Additionally, try the following visually calming activities:

- Provide novelty lights such as Lava lamps, Christmas tree lights, night lights, lights with a revolving shade that projects a soft colored picture on the wall

- Replace light bulbs with lower wattage ones or use pastel colored bulbs. Avoid fluorescent or flickering lights
- Play a simple game such as 'Peek-a-boo,' having your child take a blanket off your face. (Note: He may or may not look you in the face, but don't force it.)
- Watch DVDs or look at pictures of familiar family members making different facial expressions in order to begin to increase your child's understanding and acceptance of various facial expressions
- Decrease visually stimulating rooms (use soft lighting, muted colors, decrease clutter)
- Provide your child with simple visual tools (e.g., picture cards or photos) for familiar activities, such as a daily chart, schedule, and checklists

Calming Oral Motor Activities

Many children with autism display food selectivity, which can be related to sensory dysfunction but may also be related to oral motor issues. Because of the importance of diet for young children, it is recommended that you consult with your child's OT or SLP (Speech & Language Pathologist) before using any of the following suggestions that pertain to food:

- 'Chewy tubes' or chewing gum, if appropriate for child's age and oral motor skill level
- Sucking on popsicles, lollipops, and hard candy
- Eating crunchy foods such as chips, raw veggies, and crackers or resistive type foods such as licorice, gummy worms, and fruit roll ups
- Mouthing favorite toys (used more with younger children)
- Blowing bubbles or a pinwheel
- Sucking through a straw, especially thick liquids such as smoothies, yogurt drinks, milkshakes, or Slurpies™
- Use of a skinny straw (provides some resistance) for drinking beverages

Calming Olfactory Activities

Aromatherapy is a new avenue that is being used to help children with SPD. Certain smells are noted to be calming and others have been identified as alerting. Since children with autism often have sensory issues related to their olfactory system, move slowly and be very observant of your child's response to this type of input. Often children with SPD view certain smells as noxious, so monitor your child's reaction to strong smells such as cleaning products, perfumes, deodorants, or cigarette smoke. Be aware that your child may overreact at a party or in a cafeteria where there are too many odors bombarding his sensory system. Even subtle smells may cause a sensory overload. Try to respect this and find an area where he can go and reorganize. Consider incorporating these activities that utilize soothing scents into your child's daily routine:

- Candles, soaps, or lotions infused with calming scents such as lavender, oil of geranium, vanilla, and rose can be provided at bathtime or before bed.
- A small unlit candle or a sachet bag filled with a preferred smell (dried petals or cotton balls infused with essential oils) can be provided to your child if he is in a stressful situation.
- Place a few drops of a preferred scent in a humidifier, on a sports wrist band that can be worn, or a favorite stuffed animal.

Note: Essential oils are potent and should always be kept out of reach of children.

Organizing

Organizing techniques are used to help your child improve his ability to sort through and manage sensory information in the most advantageous fashion. They are used in an effort to maintain that calm/alert state. Calm/alert is the optimal state of arousal, which basically means your sensory system is modulated and ready to engage in fine or gross motor activities and prepared to learn. Our sensory systems unconsciously know when to calm or alert our brains in order to focus or attend to an activity. People with adequate sensory processing systems probably use many organizing strategies without even being aware, for example eating crunchy foods, sucking on a piece of hard candy, jogging, chewing on the tip of a pencil, squeezing a tennis ball, or listening to music. The sensory diet will provide your child with various types of input to keep him organized. Choose from the activities listed above to provide either calming or alerting input (depending on what the child needs) that will help him regulate his response to sensory information.

Incorporating Sensory Strategies into Everyday Activities

Don't hesitate to integrate the sensory strategies listed above into your child's daily routine during downtime, bathing, dressing, and leisure activities. It may take some time to figure out the most seamless way to do this, but trust your instincts and watch your child for signs that he's responding positively or negatively to input. Following are some suggestions for using sensory diet techniques while teaching new skills, as well as some general guidelines for making the world a more comfortable place for your child with SPD.

Bathing & Hairwashing

Warm water is naturally calming and is a nice way to end the day. Washing and drying your child with a terrycloth washcloth and towel

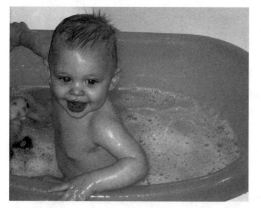

offers deep pressure. Help your child participate in bathing by soaping up a washcloth and providing hand over hand guidance (your hand on top of child's). Establish a routine with words or a rhyme (e.g., right arm up/down 1-2-3, left arm up/down 1-2-3, etc.). The deep pressure and use of a sequence may motivate your child to participate. As the practice becomes more familiar, slowly fade out your help and encourage him to continue on his own. If resistance follows, return to helping him and again slowly try to decrease hand over hand help.

Before attempting to wash your child's hair, which can be particularly difficult for some kids, make sure you have all your supplies on hand. Provide ear plugs or a waterproof visor if tolerated. Massage your child's head before hairwashing. This gives him some forewarning about what is to come next and helps him build up some tolerance for tactile input. Use tear-free or no-rinse shampoo and tangle-free conditioner, or an all-in-one product. (Try www.southpaw.com or www.drugstore.com.) Count aloud while you wash and tell him when he can expect it to be over. Rinse off by pouring water from a large cup instead of using a spray nozzle or showerhead. For children who are under-responsive to tactile input, monitor them closely in the bathtub especially if the water is too hot as they could be at risk for scalding themselves.

The use of picture charts for grooming routines is beneficial for kids with autism. Additionally, you might place similar grooming materials (hairbrush, lotion, deodorant, toothpaste) in a small container labeled with your child's name in the bathroom to aid in forming a regular routine.

Dressing

It's a good idea to use a dressing chart with either photos or drawings of clothing items in the order they are to be put on. Teaching your child to remove each picture as he dons the item will help him with sequencing the steps. Just as was described with bathing, use hand over hand help. Your child's hand should always be on the clothing article with your hand on top. As you are doing the dressing, guide his hand to help. As he becomes more compliant, wait and see if he follows through independently. As his skills and compliance increase, slowly start to decrease help. Remember, the idea is to encourage active versus passive participation.

You've probably determined by now if your child is more comfortable in tight or loose fitting clothing. Most kids prefer cotton fabrics, but some, who are tactilely defensive, like to "feel" tightness and do well with snug clothing against their body (nylon or spandex material provides ongoing deep pressure throughout the day). Remove tags from clothing or purchase clothes without tags. For undergarments, opt for socks without seams (sold by Striderite™) or tight socks, which may be easier for your child to tolerate. You can also try turning socks inside out so your child can't as easily feel the seams. For older girls, purchase all-cotton bras—avoid those with lace or underwires. Or try sports bras or cotton camisoles with built-in bras. Clothing may be more easily tolerated if it is associated with a character or color that your child likes. If possible, take your older child shopping and let him tell you what he'll wear.

Tactilely sensitive kids may have difficulty with new clothing (due to the stiffness or smell) so it's a good rule of thumb to wash new clothes a few times before asking your child to wear them. But be judicious with fabric softeners, especially if your child is sensitive to odors. When trying to desensitize your child with an article of clothing, try to slowly increase his wearing time by having him put on the item for a few minutes, and distracting him with either a preferred toy or video. Slowly try to increase the time.

To increase tolerance for wearing shoes, possibly use the brushing program (see Chapter 7 for details) or provide deep pressure to your child's feet by having him shuffle his feet across the carpet just prior to putting on shoes. Slip-on shoes or slippers may be better tolerated than hard, stiff shoes. For new shoes, break them in by stretching and bending them to loosen them up. To increase tolerance for hats or helmets, try to massage your child's head before putting these items on. For children who refuse to wear gloves or hats in the winter months, be on the lookout for frostbite.

Toothbrushing

Many children with sensory issues are resistant to toothbrushing. Some children may benefit from use of an electric toothbrush as the vibration can be calming and organizing. Initially, provide your child time to explore and experiment with his toothbrush in order to get used to it. If your child refuses to brush his teeth on his own, you will need to do the task. Always show him the toothbrush and tell him what you are doing. Again, he may benefit

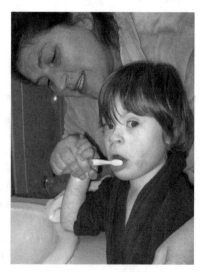

from a rhyme or counting so that he can slowly begin to increase his tolerance for the task. As tolerance begins to improve, provide some hand over hand and have him try to help you brush his teeth.

Self-Feeding

There are often many issues for children with autism and SPD surrounding eating. Resistance to food or the act of eating is not unusual. If your child has difficulty tolerating the metal of utensils (either holding the handle or having the bowl of the spoon touch his mouth or teeth), he may be more apt to use plastic utensils or those with rubber handles. If your child is still resistant to holding utensils, you may need to provide 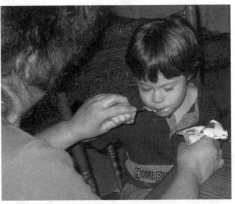 some hand over hand help by placing his hand on the spoon and your hand on top of his, while providing deep pressure. Begin this process using his favorite foods (e.g., ice cream) and decrease your help as he begins to comply. Using a suction cup bowl (especially for younger children) may help to keep the bowl in place while new feeding skills and tolerance are taught.

Eating

Many children with autism are described as picky eaters—only eating certain foods and usually refusing any new foods or textures. Some children view activities centered around the mouth as very invasive. A sensory diet can help to desensitize and improve your child's tolerance for foods and textures, but this is definitely an area where you'll need the guidance of an OT, particularly if your child has major food refusals, e.g., only eats certain textures or gags on coarser foods. An OT trained to evaluate your child's sensory issues and behavior should be able to "open the door" by slowly introducing certain tastes and techniques that you can use at home. Many children with food issues prefer very bland foods but may actually respond well to odd tastes, such as sour candies, salsa, and so on. Often, these odd food tastes can help "wake up" the mouth. Following such input, the child may begin to show increased curiosity and

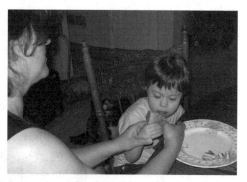

accept new foods and textures. This input is always presented very slowly, with the therapist carefully looking for the "alert" moment.

Toileting

Many children with autism have difficulty with toileting. This can be due to many reasons, e.g., a control issue, which may require a behavior-based approach. If you suspect your child's difficulty with toilet training stems from sensory issues, consider the following reasons and recommendations. Perhaps he is upset by the sound, volume, or suddenness of a flushing toilet. To increase tolerance for this auditory stimulation, have him help to flush the toilet while you count or recite a fun rhyme or song. Your child may also be fearful of sitting on the toilet seat. Provide a small child's potty chair or, if he is too big for one, purchase a toilet ring reducer and provide a small stool to support his feet so he is aware of where his body is in space. Children who are under-responsive may not be aware when their diaper is wet or messy. Start by teaching the concepts of wet and dry by letting him feel the difference between wet and dry washcloths. When taking off a dirty diaper, have your child feel the diaper and tell you if it is wet or dry.

Toilet training a child who is autistic can be complicated and may require more strategies than the ones listed in this book. Additional resources for toilet training are provided in the Resource section of this book.

Bedtime Routine

Many parents report that getting their child to settle down for bed is a difficult task. Establishing a predictable bedtime routine is essential. Consider incorporating some of the following calming sensory techniques:

- A warm bath with soothing lavender body wash
- Deep pressure, i.e., a back massage or rubbing the body with lotion
- Soft calming music
- Looking at books or listening to music while rocking in a rocking chair
- Heavy blankets tucked firmly around the child's body
- Large body pillows or stuffed animals wedged close to the child's body
- A Lava lamp or lights that project shadows on the ceiling or walls

Chores

Household chores are an excellent source of providing "heavy work," which can be organizing to the sensory system. Chores will not only prove a beneficial ingredient in your child's sensory diet but will help your child be a contributing member of the family. Remember, with all of these tasks, you will initially need to provide hand over hand help and step-by-step instruction to increase both compliance and success with the task. The following is a list of everyday jobs that may work for your child:

- Pushing a child-sized shopping cart in the grocery store
- Locating grocery items while shopping, either with words or pictures of items
- Helping to put away groceries (stacking cans, carrying items to the pantry)
- Helping to push trash cans to the curb
- Pushing or pulling a wagon full of recyclable cans or newspapers
- Ripping up junk mail
- Carrying a laundry basket full of clothes
- Pushing chairs under the table after eating
- Washing the car
- Dusting furniture
- Squirting or watering plants
- Setting or clearing the table

- Wiping off the table
- Feeding pets
- Brushing pets
- Walking a dog
- Raking leaves
- Sweeping
- Vacuuming

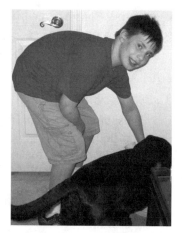

Play and Leisure Activities

Many children with autism exhibit odd play skills. They may line up their toys or play with an object in a perseverative manner. Some of these behaviors are related to autism but some will likely be due to poor sensory processing, e.g., intolerance to holding objects in hands. You will need to be very observant as to what type of sensory information your child may be seeking or avoiding. He may only want to focus on one aspect of a toy, e.g., hitting the same button to hear a particular sound over and over. You may need to walk him through the steps of how to play appropriately with the toy by providing hand over hand help. This may or may not work since the specific action that your child is engaging in may be part of a self-stimulatory behavior (related more to autism). This is when you may need to find other types of sensory input (deep pressure, visual, auditory, etc.) that may decrease the need for self-stimming.

As far as leisure activities, many kids with SPD benefit from the sensory input that sports and outdoor activities provide, i.e., gymnastics, karate, swimming, running, dancing, hiking, bike riding, etc. Some kids will enjoy team sports or group activities that focus on the experience itself rather than competition, while others (who have autism and SPD) might want to consider competing in the Special Olympics.

Out in the Community

The world around us is an ever-changing environment. Many children with autism can handle their own familiar surroundings but fall apart in unfamiliar settings. It is essential that you observe your child's body language in response to a new environment. Children may have difficulty tolerating all the sensory information (odors, sounds, visual stimuli) in the environment and lose control. Your child may benefit from listening to preferred music over earphones or soft ear plugs to muffle noise. Your child might react to all of the visual stimulation and you may need to locate a darkened or less stimulating area of the environment where he can retreat. But this may not always be possible, such as if you are at the circus or a ballgame, and this is where tried and true sensory strategies may help, e.g., drinking through a straw, or chewing crunchy foods or gummy candies. Be aware that even with these strategies in your arsenal you may need to have a back up plan such as taking your child out of the room and walking him around or rocking him until he is able to calm down.

What Outcome Can I Expect from Regular Use of a Sensory Diet?

As your child begins to realize that the sensory diet is helping, you should begin to notice that he is able to use these strategies *on himself* during his daily routine. His independence and functional skills should increase. Your child's desire for tactile input though vibration might take the form of using the mixer to help you make a cake. Ripping up junk mail that provides deep pressure may result in increased hand strength for holding a pen and writing. The use of headphones might enable him to tolerate auditory stimulation and calm him for sleep. Rolling on the floor first thing in the morning might alert his system to attend to getting dressed. Supervised roughhousing might increase your child's interaction and participation with his siblings. Hopefully he will have less hypersensitivity to things like food and clothing.

Additionally, you may also notice a decrease in self-stimulatory behaviors. Your child might still engage in them but with use of a scheduled sensory diet and sensory activities, he will likely be less engaged in stimming behaviors. In the case of an aggressive child or one who exhibits self-injurious behaviors, hopefully you'll see a decrease in those behaviors as well. These changes will positively affect your child's relationships with family and peers. The increase in your child's level of calm alertness will positively affect his ability to participate and learn at school, home, and in the community.

Your child's sensory diet provides structure for the family and use of a chart or diary will provide a concrete outline in order to determine what is or is not working. Since you will be an active participant in developing the sensory diet (times and types of activities needed throughout the day), you will become a more vigilant observer of your child's behavior and his response to input. More than likely you will begin to have lots of ideas and be able to share them with your child's OT during future visits. The bottom line is that once you begin to feel comfortable, the diet will continue to develop more from your input than that of the OT. How long your child is on the diet will depend on how much input he needs or when his sensory system is able to tell him "when and how much." Ideally, your child will reach the goal of actively engaging in these sensory techniques independently throughout his day.

Conclusion

Above is a sampling of activities that might become part of your child's sensory diet. It would be nice if you could provide the same sensory diet for every child with SPD, but alas, each child's needs vary. Working with an experienced occupational therapist trained in a sensory-based approach to establish your child's sensory diet is your first step. The activities recommended are to be used throughout your child's day and will provide him with small or large doses of sensory input, whatever is needed at that exact time (determined by you and your observation of his behaviors during the day). Become very observant of your child's reaction to the techniques and work slowly at building up a daily sensory routine that works best for your child and your family. All of these sensory experiences will begin to improve your child's ability to make sense of input in order to reach that calm/alert state, which is the optimal time to teach your child new skills. If some behaviors persist and are getting in the way of learning, the sensory work you have done may provide the framework for using behavioral strategies that may further improve his compliance with daily tasks.

By now, you realize that this is a slow, but hopefully steady process towards improving your child's ability to make sense of incoming sensory input. Keep in mind that sensory needs can change and the efficacy of your child's diet will need to be frequently reassessed. Ongoing therapy sessions will help to tailor your child's sensory diet and provide more precise activities that will help him calm during stressful times and alert during downtime.

10 Sensory Strategies in the School Environment

We have spent a great deal of time examining how a poor sensory processing system can affect your child's ability to function in everyday activities. If your child has sensory processing issues, you're hopefully using a sensory diet and setting up the home environment to suit his needs. But what about school? Our kids spend a lot of time at school—a very stimulating environment. Imagine a kindergarten classroom with twenty kids all running around, talking loudly, playfully bumping into each other, hanging up their coats, pulling out paint, markers, and glue. Likely, the room is bright with boldly colored charts to help motivate the children. There are probably different areas for free play. Maybe there is an overhead PA system and bells or alarms for the older children who change classes. Now try to imagine how a child with a poor sensory processing system is going to deal with all of this input. Remember, in order for a child to learn or focus on an activity, he must be able to modulate or regulate all of the incoming sensory input in an appropriate manner in order to achieve the "just right" level. This won't be easy for a child with a sensory processing disorder and as a result he'll likely engage in behaviors that will distract his teachers and classmates and negatively affect his ability to learn.

The educational setting chosen for a child with ASD and a sensory processing disorder can run the gamut. A child who is non-verbal may be in a self-contained classroom. A child with Asperger's disorder may be mainstreamed into a general education classroom with an aide. Regardless of their school placement or level of cognitive development, children in either of these scenarios can benefit from the use of sensory strategies at school. From the examples below we can see how simply rearranging the environment and using sensory strategies can greatly improve the chances that these kids will find the "just right" level to regulate their sensory systems and begin to focus on classroom tasks. (More detailed case studies are explored later in this chapter.)

Kenny (who was introduced in Chapter 5) is non-verbal, over-responsive to sounds, tactile input, and movement. He is considered a "sensory avoider." Kenny is in a self-contained classroom with five other children, one teacher, and an aide.
Problem: *Kenny screams when it is time to sit on the floor for story time.*
Strategy:
  Environment—*Kenny is moved to a slightly darkened area of the room, where he can still see and hear the teacher tell the story, but is further away from the other children.*
  Sensory Approach—*To address his oversensitivity, Kenny is seated in a bean bag chair (provides deep pressure), given a few small toys that provide tactile and deep pressure, a small bag of crunchy or chewy foods, such as pretzels and gummy worms (provide heavy work to the mouth), and soft ear plugs (to muffle some of the background noises).*
Outcome: *The sensory strategies and altered environment allow Kenny to feel calmer and be able to listen to the story at the same time as the other children.*

Kayla (who was introduced in Chapter 5) has Asperger's disorder, is highly verbal, and is included in a general education classroom. She is under-responsive to movement and tactile input. She is over-responsive to sound.
Problem: *Kayla talks too loud and runs around the classroom, bumping into furniture, during the time she is supposed to be learning her spelling words. Spelling is always after the morning announcements on the PA and a bell usually rings about fifteen minutes thereafter for a class change.*
Strategy:
  Environment—*Before the morning announcements, Kayla is directed to a quiet "chill-out" area of the room, with decreased visual and auditory stimulation.*
  Sensory Approach—*Kayla is provided ear plugs, which still allow her to hear voices, but muffles background sounds and*

the noise from the overhead PA system. She is seated at a small desk on a wiggle cushion, which allows her to move around while seated. She is given playdough and letter cut-outs, which provide deep pressure when she rolls out the dough and pushes in the cookie cutter letters to complete her spelling words.

Outcome: *The sensory strategies and altered environment allow Kayla to have increased visual alertness to focus on the task of spelling her words. When necessary, she is given quiet cues from her aide to make up sentences with the spelled out words.*

Just as it is important to utilize sensory strategies and a sensory diet at home, it is also essential that it is carried over in the school environment, where the child's optimal level of alertness is necessary for learning to take place. Teachers are liable to have many questions regarding how this approach can be integrated into the school environment and schedule. Refer to the list of list of simple "Do's and Don'ts" in Chapter 9 and below for answers to common questions school personnel are likely to have.

How is the sensory diet set up at school?

Your child's sensory diet may initially be set up by the school occupational therapist (OT). The OT will observe the student within the classroom setting and interview the teacher and other staff members who are directly involved with your child or student regarding what behaviors are getting in the way of learning. The OT will evaluate the student using different types of sensory strategies and noting his response to the input. If possible, the OT will contact the student's family, especially if they are using a sensory diet at home. Sensory strategies that are successful at home may be able to be used during the school day. Once all the information is gathered, the school OT should set up the following guidelines:

- Adjust the classroom environment accordingly, i.e., providing a quiet "chill-out" area, decreasing visual or auditory stimuli, etc. (See Environment section below.)
- Set up a schedule to use the sensory diet at specified times of the day, e.g., 9:00AM— ear plugs; 10:00AM— small fidgets in hands during a lesson; 11:00AM—erase

the blackboard (heavy work) for alerting and organizing to focus on a math lesson.

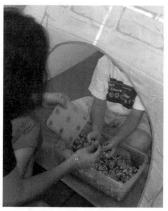

- Train staff (teacher or aide) to use the sensory strategies and explain their purpose.
- If possible, involve the student in the use of sensory strategies and make him more aware of how and when to use them, along with why they help.
- Regularly monitor the student in different school environments, e.g., cafeteria, playground, etc. to see how the diet is working.
- Regular follow-up with staff as to what is working and what needs to be adjusted.

Environment

Environment and setting are important factors in the success of a sensory diet. Below is a list of suggestions to help modify the student's school surroundings. Some may not always be appropriate, depending on the age and school placement (inclusion versus a mainstreamed classroom setting; preschool versus middle school). However, they may provide you with some ideas about how or where you may be able to adapt.

- Much like you would at home, provide a "chill-out" area in the classroom where there is less "traffic," both visual and auditory. This becomes a "safe" area where a student can go to regroup. The area might be somewhat darkened, have a bean bag chair to provide deep pressure to the child, a small box of fidgets (stress balls, squeeze toys), soft background music (calming or classical), crunchy or chewy foods (pretzels, gummy worms, licorice), and soft lighting, such as Christmas lights or a Lava lamp. If a "chill-out" area is not appropriate or simply not feasible, determine some area within the school that the student can go when he needs to regroup such as a small room, little closet, nurse's station where there is limited visual or auditory distracters.

- For a younger, tactilely defensive child who needs physical space, delineate a separate area for him to sit on, such as a carpet tile, a beanbag chair, or a space on the carpet bordered by masking tape.
- Provide a designated area for personal belongings.
- Provide a wiggle cushion or oversized therapy ball for sensory seeking children to sit on during times they are expected to focus on an activity.

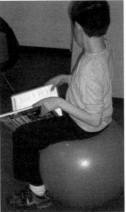

- Decrease glaring or excessively bright lighting (fluorescent lights, sunny window area) if possible.
- Allow the child with SPD to take tests in a separate room (to reduce distractions) or provide extra time if they are slow to process visual information.
- Provide checklists for daily activities or assignments on the classroom wall or taped to the student's desk. If the student can write, begin to help him write up his own schedule on paper or on the computer.
- Use visual supports (e.g., picture cards, timers) and other cues to help with organization and the daily schedule so that the student is more aware of time, transitions, and changes in routine.

Who carries out the sensory diet within the school environment?

Up until this point, your student has likely been engaging in self-stimulation to deal with SPD and those behaviors might not be appropriate in the school setting or conducive to learning. In the beginning, before the routine has been established, someone should initiate and monitor sensory activities. Once the diet has been set up, it will need to be carried out throughout the day. Ideally, this can be done by your student's aide. If your child has no aide then he is likely self-sufficient enough to take cues from his teacher or a picture schedule, chart, or checklist to follow the diet.

As a school OT, do I need to have special certification to set up a sensory diet?

No specific certification is needed. However, good, solid knowledge of sensory processing is essential in order to develop a sensory diet and use sensory strategies effectively. There are many weekend courses offered by OTs who specialize in sensory processing and issues related to children with autism. OTs can usually find a list of courses by contacting The American Occupational Therapy Association, Inc. (AOTA), looking at websites, or professional magazines that may have information about continuing education courses on this subject. (A potentially helpful list of resources is provided at the end of this book.)

How is the sensory diet carried out at school?

Many sensory strategies for calming, alerting, and organizing your child's sensory system were laid out in Chapter 9. Most of these techniques can be adapted for use in the school environment. If not, you can experiment to find activities that follow the same principles and are age-appropriate and conducive to the classroom. Below are some ideas that work in a school setting for calming, alerting, and organizing.

General:

- Help your student create his own customized sensory bag. Fill a backpack or fanny pack that can travel with him throughout the school day with items that help him calm or organize, e.g., crunchy foods, ear plugs, squishy toy, scented sachet.
- Try to incorporate sensory input into a functional task. For example, if your student needs help to alert, you might suggest he do something physical, like hand out books, or be in charge of the roll call by crossing off each child's name on the blackboard.

- Think "outside the box." Children with autism often have a fascination with specific subjects or activities. Using these as motivators and applying sensory techniques will help the student focus and attend to a task. For example, with a tactilely defensive child who refuses to hold a marker but loves playdough, use playdough as a medium for teaching. Bury objects in the playdough and 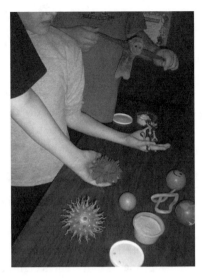 have the student find them and count them, match them, add and subtract them. Use cookie cutters to press letters out of playdough to spell words. The playdough provides deep pressure and good tactile input.

Alerting:

- Teachers can provide "action breaks" and opportunities for "heavy work" before academics or demanding tasks. (See Heavy Work Activities below.) These might include jumping jacks, hopping on one foot, spinning in place five times, relay races from one end of room to other, handing out books.
- Teachers can change the pitch of their voice (loud, animated, whisper), or sing or rhyme directions in order to alert their students' auditory sense.
- Students can hold fidgets or use vibrating pens during lesson times.
- Teachers can use concrete manipulatives to teach concepts.
- Students can keep a sachet of an alerting scent in their desks.
- Students can chew on a straw or chewy tube or drink water through a sports bottle during study time.
- Students and teachers can organize work using brightly colored folders.

Calming:

- Teachers can speak with a calming voice and use simple words at a slower pace.
- Teachers can seat a sensitive student away from noise and bright light (windows, chatty children).
- Teachers can make sure the sensitive child has extra personal space in a group and can assign him job of line leader or line ender or door holder.
- Teachers should approach the over-responsive student from the front and use deep, firm pressure versus light touch if contact is necessary.
- Students can keep a sachet of a calming scent in their desks, or put on scented chapstick, or a few drops of essential oil on a terrycloth wristband.
- Students can wear weighted vests or use weighted pencils and spoons.
- Teachers can warn student in advance of fire drills or bells ringing for class changes.
- Teachers may need to provide reminders to students to go to the "chill-out" area for five minutes to decompress.

Heavy Work Activities:

Heavy work is mostly proprioceptive input and provides deep pressure. Heavy work activities have been found to help the student improve modulation by allowing the sensory system to calm or alert (depending on what that particular needs). Optimal modulation will allow the brain to organize and improve the student's ability to focus and attend to a task. Below is a list of some heavy work activities that could easily be integrated into a school sensory diet.

- Erasing chalkboards
- Washing desks
- Pushing or moving desks or stacking books
- Stapling papers
- Emptying wastebaskets
- Pulling blinds or shades up or down
- Pushing milk cart in cafeteria
- Bringing lunches from the cafeteria
- Handing out snacks or drinks

- Sharpening pencils
- Ripping up old papers
- Using the paper shredder (supervised)
- Tying a Thera-Band® around the front legs of a chair and allowing the student to kick his feet
- Pulling on Thera-Band® tied to the side of a chair
- Gardening or watering plants with a squirt bottle
- Running around a track
- Wood shop or wood projects, requiring hammering, sanding, or painting
- Scheduling art or gym class before a sit-down subject such as math
- Wheelbarrel walks
- Jumping rope or follow the leader-type games
- Any recess or gym activity

As a school OT, how do I find the time to set up a sensory diet for a particular student?

School OTs usually have a pretty extensive caseload. Finding the time and resources to set up a sensory diet can be challenging. To save time, the school OT should touch base with the school staff and the student's parents to determine what the student's sensory needs are. If the child is receiving the services of a private OT, the school OT can consult with her (with the parent's permission) regarding what they've been working on. Private OTs usually have the luxury of working one on one with a child for at least an hour per week. They are provided more quality time to explore and determine optimal sensory strategies. They also tend to have more face to face contact with the parent. Most private OTs will be more than willing to share their ideas about which strategies to incorporate into the student's school program.

Will use of a sensory diet interfere with a student's behavioral intervention plan?

The use of a regular sensory diet should actually complement a student's behavioral intervention program. As we have noted throughout this book, children with autism often demonstrate a variety of challenging behaviors. Those behaviors motivated by sensory needs should be addressed by a sensory diet and those that are related more to autism will best be addressed through use of a behavioral protocol. It will be very important that the school OT works in conjunction with the behavioral therapist and that use of a sensory diet be established within the behavioral protocol.

How will I know if all this effort is making a difference for the student?

Since not all behaviors that children with autism and sensory problems display are related to SPD, it can be tricky to determine how much affect the sensory diet is having. However, if your student

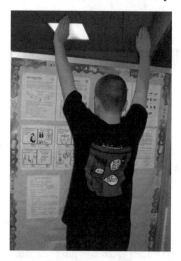

is having difficulty with an activity, and after being provided with sensory input is able to comply or attend to the task, then the behavior is more than likely related to difficulty with sensory processing. The beauty of using a sensory diet is that if the sensory strategy you're using is working, then the particular behavior you're focusing on will be improved or extinguished, and other behaviors (not related to SPD) can then be addressed using a behavioral approach.

Ultimately, the goal is for the student to be able to perform sensory strategies on himself. Ideally, your student will carry with him a customized sensory bag or have a small box in his desk or backpack that contains some sensory items (e.g., hand fidgets, stress balls, pretzels, ear plugs). He'll use these during the school day, or engage in some heavy work tasks, or retreat to the "chill-out" area of the room as needed. He may also be directed to a visual chart of sensory diet strategies that he can carry out independently.

Case Studies

The case studies and charts that follow illustrate how an OT observes various behaviors in children with sensory issues, sets up a sensory diet and schedule, and provides specific sensory strategies that enable them to increase tolerance and compliance for cooperation and learning. Keep in mind, there is no single cookbook approach that works. Every child will display a specific set of behaviors unique to only them. And as children become older, some activities such as using a swing, ball, or trampoline may not be available or appropriate to the school setting. It will be the job of the school staff or OT to determine what types of sensory strategies are suitable for the particular environment. Using the suggestions in this chapter and the previous one, along with constant observation of the child's response should help you carry out a sensory diet within the school environment.

Jahmal

Jahmal is an eight-year-old boy who was diagnosed with autism at the age of three. He understands simple commands and uses a few words to communicate. At school he communicates using picture exchange cards. Jahmal attends a private school in a self-contained classroom with a special education teacher, one aide, and five other children with autism. Jahmal loves playing video games on the computer. He is also fascinated with spelling words but refuses to write or draw.

He displays many behaviors in response to his many sensory issues, including constantly getting up and moving around the room, and holding his ears or tilting his ear to his shoulder in an effort to block out noise. Because he hates tags in his clothing and wearing new clothes, he often tries to remove his clothes during the day. He will provide eye contact but does not visually attend or focus on an activity. This is affecting his eye-hand skills and overall learning. Jahmal also has many behaviors that are disruptive to the class. One such behavior involves putting one foot in front of the other and rocking back and forth in place. While doing this he usually flaps his hands over his ears or in front of his face. He also tends to clap his hands and make guttural noises.

His teacher notes that being in constant motion seems to help Jahmal focus and attend to many of the lessons. While he is seated in his chair, his teacher also notes that he often tips the chair onto the back legs and then drops the chair forward, back onto the all four legs. This again makes a great deal of noise and is distracting. Following lunch or activities in the gym or auditorium, he seems generally more "out of control" (running around the room, stimming on hands, or making silly noises).

Jahmal receives occupational therapy and behavioral services as part of his school program. Services are usually provided directly within his classroom. Jahmal also has been receiving private outpatient services for the past year. His OT has been helping to develop a sensory diet for home use, along with improving his ability to increase participation in daily activities such as dressing, grooming, getting a snack or drink, and increasing his leisure skills repertoire. His school OT has been in contact with both the private therapist and Jahmal's parents in an effort to transition some successful sensory strategies to the classroom setting. Problem behaviors were identified by school staff, the behavioral therapist, and the school OT, and a chart was developed listing concerns and possible solutions.

Jahmal still faces many issues, but identifying and providing sensory strategies to address his sensory needs has helped improve many of his behaviors and he is showing more tolerance and compliance within his classroom. (Refer to chart on pages 164-66.) Obviously, more sensory strategies can be used in his self-contained classroom than in a typical classroom setting. For comparison, below is the case study of a child who is mainstreamed into an inclusive classroom.

Stephen

Stephen is a thirteen-year-old boy with Asperger's disorder. He has a high IQ and is very verbal. He loves composing stories (but not writing them down) and playing video games. Up through last year, Stephen was included in mainstream classes until ongoing behavioral issues warranted his removal. Specifically, he was often moving about the classroom, doing karate moves, purposely banging his body into walls, and kicking the rungs of his chair or the student's chair in front of him. He needed constant reminders to sit down. Other distracting behaviors included humming, talking aloud, and fidgeting during sit-down tasks. At various times of the day, Stephen was acting either very keyed up or very sleepy. He was also noncompliant with handwriting tasks but was usually more cooperative when allowed to type on the computer.

Stephen tends to be very concrete in his thinking and gets upset when teachers try to help him to understand abstract thoughts. He has difficulty understanding other people's body language and facial expressions, and the concept of personal space. He becomes upset if anyone tries to correct his behavior and he often cannot tell when someone is upset with him.

His grooming skills are poor and his hair is often dirty and unkempt. He prefers to wear well-worn clothing that is often too small. These issues are becoming more troublesome as Stephen enters puberty and his peers are beginning to make fun of him. His parents report that at home he has a very hard time getting going in the morning and needs constant cues to perform hygiene skills.

Due to ongoing issues, Stephen has been attending classes in the resource room. His OT, behavioral therapist, and special education teacher are working together to determine what types of sensory input will help Stephen alert and attend without distracting everyone else in the classroom. A daily schedule was developed and is outlined below.

Although Jahmal and Stephen are at opposite ends of the autism spectrum, they both have something in common—sensory process disorder. By determining their individual strengths and weaknesses, their occupational therapists have been able to provide each a tailor-made sensory diet. (Refer to chart on pages 167-69.) Use of the diet will help provide the "just right" input in order for each child to more actively participate in school. This process will address sensory needs and involve use of behavioral strategies and consistent communication between home and school. The result will be better sensory processing and a more engaged student who is ready to learn.

Jahmal

Behavioral Concerns	Sensory Need	Possible Solutions	Functional Outcome
Rocking on feet in a standing position	Seeking vestibular and proprioceptive input	■ Bounce on small trampoline in back of room (supervised by aide) ■ Sit or bounce on a therapy ball (supervised by aide) ■ Five minutes of jumping and running before beginning lessons ■ A heavy work activity five minutes before lessons begin	Engaging in movement activities fulfills Jahmal's vestibular and proprioceptive needs before lessons and enables him to focus on the lesson without disturbing other students.
Flapping hands over ears and eyes	Possibly trying to decrease the amount of visual or auditory input (due to difficulty blocking out visual stimuli and background noises)	■ Seat in a quieter or less visual distracting part of the classroom ■ Provide soft ear plugs	Reducing some of the excessive stimulation to his eyes and ears decreases Jahmal's flapping. However, he will still do this if he is overwhelmed by events of the day.
Balancing chair on back legs and pitching forward	Seeking vestibular and proprioceptive input in response to the movement of the chair	■ Sitting in a rocking chair (supervised by aide) ■ Thera-Band tied to the sides of chair, which Jahmal can pull on, providing him with some resistance ■ Thera-Band placed on the rungs of his chair, which Jahmal can push and pull with his legs, providing resistance	The rocking chair provides Jahmal with the vestibular and proprioceptive input he craves and helps him focus and attend to activities. The Thera-Band activities provide resistance, or heavy work, which also help him organize and focus.

Making guttural noises	Providing himself with auditory feedback or attempting to block out background noises	■ Chewing on resistive products (chewy tube, crunchy or chewy foods) ■ Sucking drinks through a sports bottle ■ Using headphones with calming or preferred music during appropriate times of the day	These first activities provide heavy work to the mouth and will help with calming and organizing the brain. Chewing and music will also provide organizing auditory feedback.
Removing clothing	Responding to tactile defensiveness with clothing and tags	■ Encourage parents to remove tags and wash clothes to soften them up ■ Encourage parents to purchase tight clothing for Jahmal to wear under school clothes ■ Develop a behavioral protocol for not removing clothes	The tighter and less distracting clothing helps calm him and decreases his temptation to remove his clothes during the school day. A behavioral protocol allows him to increase compliance and earn rewards.
Acting "out of control" following lunch and activities in gym or auditorium	Overstimulated by large spaces and too much noise	■ Provide five-ten minutes in the "chill-out" area following lunch or "big room" activities to help Jahmal regroup	The absence of stimulation allows Jahmal to calm his sensory system before he needs to sit and focus on school tasks.

(Continued on next page.)

(Continued from previous page.)

Avoiding sit-down tasks, especially hand-writing	Visual motor skills are poor and too many sensory demands are likely affecting compliance	■ Capitalizing on his love of letters and spelling, use stickers to match letters on paper or place magnetic letters on a metal file cabinet ■ Provide a vibrating pen to get attention and focus on paper-work	Jahmal responds well to movement and novelty. His love of spelling is also being incorporated into the task but not necessarily using a pencil at this time. He is still working on increasing his tolerance for holding a pencil but novel ideas such as writing letters in sand, shaving cream, etc. are being used. The computer is also being used with various games.
Holding ears or tilting ear to shoulder in response to loud noises	Trying to decrease auditory stimulation due to hypersensitivity	■ Provide headphones when appropriate ■ Provide soft ear plugs ■ When possible provide warning about when to expect loud noises	Using headphones or soft ear plugs has cut down significantly on this behavior. Jahmal is also provided a chart of activities to expect throughout the day, including times when overhead alarms will go off.
Constantly moving; difficulty sitting down during lessons	Seeking proprioceptive and vestibular input	■ Sitting on a wiggle cushion ■ Allowing Jahmal to do heavy work (e.g., handing out papers, books, wiping chalk board) ■ Developing a behavioral protocol with rewards for sitting following movement activities	Use of heavy work and sitting on a wiggle cushion or rocking chair have significantly helped Jahmal sit for some of his lessons. Also, use of the behavioral protocol is helping him to tolerate longer periods of time seated at a desk or table.

Stephen

Behavioral Concerns	Sensory Need	Possible Solutions	Functional Outcome
Getting out of his seat and constantly moving	Seeking vestibular input	■ Provide a seat in the back of the room and a designated space to stand up and move around ■ Provide a wiggle cushion that allows him to move a bit while seated ■ OT and Behavioral therapist develop a list of rules about inappropriate classroom behavior	Providing a separate area at the back of the room where he can provide his own sensory input without disturbing the class has enabled Stephen to return to his regular classroom. Following behavior rules earns him points for special preferred activities.
Standing up and doing karate moves	Seeking proprioceptive input	■ Stationary bike and large body pillows are provided in the resource room ■ Thera-Bands on the sides of his classroom chair to pull for resistance ■ Doing push ups against the back wall of classroom ■ Squeezing fidgets in his pockets ■ Five minutes of jumping or running exercises before going to class	Stephen spends some time in the resource room where he can get more sensory input via the bike or rolling on large body pillows, but this extra input allows him to spend most of his time in the classroom. Any additional sensory input he needs he is able to carry out in the regular class without disturbing others.

(Continued on next page.)

(Continued from previous page.)

Constantly fidgeting and making noises	Seeking proprioceptive and auditory feedback	■ OT provides Stephen's teachers with a list of heavy work activities that can be done before a lesson, e.g., ripping up old papers, wiping chalkboards, getting out supplies for lesson	Heavy work not only helps him to organize before a lesson, but the activities also help to increase his interaction and participation within the classroom.
Acting either "wired" or very sleepy	Difficulty with sensory modulation and getting his sensory system at the "just right" level for learning	■ Using the "Alert Program" chart, which has low, high, and "just right" categories. The school OT has taught Stephen to determine where he feels his sensory system is, and the chart then directs him to choose from different types of sensory strategies to alert or calm his sensory system accordingly	This system lets Stephen determine what types of sensory input he needs to help modulate his sensory system independently.
Poor grooming skills and insistence to wear well-worn clothing that is very small	hypersensitivity to textures (tactile)	■ Following a checklist for grooming tasks (e.g., brushing teeth, putting on deodorant, washing hair on Monday and Wednesday, etc.). ■ Family determines which clothes are too small and need to be thrown away	Completion of his hygiene checklist on a daily basis earns him extra time on the computer playing video games. School and home working together help Stephen continue to improve his daily living skills and prepare him for more independence as an adult.

		■ New clothing purchased with Stephen's input and washed many times before he is expected to wear it ■ Attending a weekly social skills group where these issues are discussed	Stephen responds well to simple cause and effect and has done well with increasing compliance to finish school activities. If he completes his checklists, he earns points for special preferred activities. By using the computer, he is more readily able to demonstrate his skills.
Non-compliance with school tasks	Visual motor skills are poor and too many sensory demands are likely affecting compliance	■ OT and Behavioral therapist create a checklist of school tasks that need to be completed in a specific time frame ■ More computer time for written work as Stephen is very bright and his handwriting skills are still very immature	

Sensory screening tests and profiles that may be used during a sensory evaluation

Assessment Tool	Author	Age-range	Description
Test of Visual–Motor Skills-revised	Gardner, 1995	3-13.11 years	Evaluates visual motor (eye hand) control to copy items
VMI—Developmental Test of Visual-Motor Integration	Beery-Butkenica, 1997	2-15 years	Divided into 3 parts (timed and un-timed). Evaluates visual motor control to copy design and visual perceptual skills to locate correct stimulus
Peabody Development of Motor Skill (PDMS-2)	Folio, Fewell (2000)	Birth – 83 months	Evaluates early childhood motor development in both gross and fine motor functioning
Movement Assessment Battery for Children (Movement) ABC	Henderson, Sugden, 1992	4-12 years divided into 4 age bands	Identifies and evaluates movement difficulties in children
Bruininks-Oseretsky Test of Motor Proficiency	Bruininks, 1978	4.5-14.5 years	Evaluates speed and performance of gross and fine motor skills through a variety of simple timed and untimed tests
De Gangi-Berk Test of Sensory Integration	DeGangi and Berk, 1983	3-5 years	Measures sensory integration along with postural control, reflex integra-tion, and bilateral motor control

SIPT—Sensory Integration and Praxis Tests	Ayres, 1989	4-8.11 years	Consists of 17 subtests that evaluate tactile, visual, and kinesthetic performance. Evaluator must be SIPT certified to give this test.
Sensory Profile	Dunn, 1999	5-10 years	Profile is filled out by the caregiver and consists of 125 items broken into 3 groups that looks at sensory modulation, processing, and emotional response in 9 areas of functioning (e.g., auditory, tactile, etc.)
Sensory Integration Inventory-Revised	Reisman, Hanschu, 1992	14-adult	Set up as an inventory that consists of 111 items divided into 4 sections (tactile, vestibular, proprioceptive, and general response)

Bibliography and Recommended Reading

American Occupational Therapy Association. (2002). Occupational therapy practice framework: Domain and Process. *American Journal of Occupational Therapy, 56,* 609-639.

American Psychiatric Association. (1994). *Diagnostic and Statistical Manual of Mental Disorders (DSM-IV),* 4th ed. Washington, DC: American Psychiatric Association.

Anderson, E. & P. Emmons. (1996). *Unlocking the Mysteries of Sensory Integration.* Arlington, TX: Future Horizons.

Anderson, W., S. Chitwood, D. Hayden & C.Takemoto. (2008). *Negotiating the Special Education Maze: A Guide for Parents and Teachers,* 4th ed. Bethesda, MD: Woodbine House.

Audet, L.R. (2003). *Teach Me How to Do It Myself: A Cognitive Self-Talk Approach to Problem Solving.* Paper presented at the biannual convention of the Ohio Autism Society, Toledo.

Ayres, A.J. (1979; revised 2005). *Sensory Integration and the Child: Understanding Hidden Sensory Challenges.* Los Angeles, CA: Western Psychological Services.

Ayres, A.J. (1972). *Sensory Integration and Learning Disorders.* Los Angeles, CA: Western Psychological Services.

Ayres, A.J. (1988). *Sensory Integration and Praxis Tests (SIPT) Manual.* Los Angeles, CA: Western Psychological Services.

Ayres, A.J. & L.S. Tickle. (1980). Hyper-responsivity to touch and vestibular stimuli as a predictor of positive response to sensory integration procedures by autistic children. *American Journal of Occupational Therapy, 34*, 375-81.

Beery, K.E. & N.A. Butkenica. (1997). *Developmental Test of Visual Motor Integration: Administration and Scoring Manual.* Parsippany, NJ: Modern Curriculum Press.

Berg, W.K. & K.M. Berg. (1979). Psychophysiological development in infancy: State, sensory function, and attention. In J. Osofsky (Ed.), *Handbook of Infant Development* (pp. 238-317). New York, NY: J. Wiley and Sons.

Biel, L. & N. Peske. (2005). *Raising a Sensory Smart Child: The Definitive Handbook for Helping Your Child with Sensory Integration Issues.* New York, NY: Penguin.

Bissell, J., J. Fisher, C. Owens & P. Polcyn. (1998). *Sensory Motor Handbook: A Guide for Implementing and Modifying Activities in the Classroom* (2nd ed). Torrence, CA: Sensory Integration International.

Blanche, E., T. Botticelli & M. Hallway (1998). *Combining Neuro-Developmental Treatment and Sensory Integration Principles: An Approach to Pediatric Therapy.* San Antonio, TX: Therapy Skill Builders.

Blanche, E. & R. Schaaf. (2001). "Proprioception: A cornerstone for sensory integrative intervention." In Roley, S., Blanche, E., & Schaaf, R. (Eds), *Understanding the Nature of Sensory Integration with Diverse Populations* (pp. 109-122). San Antonio, TX: The Psychological Corporation.

Brazelton, T.B., E. Tronick, L. Adamson, H. Als & S. Wise. (1975). Early mother-infant reciprocity. In M.A. Hofer (Ed.), *The Parent-Infant Relationship* (pp. 137-155). London: Ciba.

Bruininks, R.H. (1978). *Bruininks-Oseretsky Test of Motor Proficiency, Examiner's Manual.* Circle Pines, MN: American Guidance Service.

Bundy, A., A. Fisher, E. Murray & S. Lane (2002). *Sensory Integration: Theory and Practice.* Philadelphia, PA: F.A. Davis.

Capone, G., M. Grados, W. Kaufmann, S. Bernad-Ripoll & A. Jewell. (2005). Down syndrome and comorbid autism spectrum disorder: Characterization using the aberrant behavior checklist. *American Journal of Medical Genetics Part A, 134A*, 373-380.

Cermak, S. (1991). Somatodyspraxia. In Fisher, A., E. Murray & A. Bundy (Eds.), *Sensory Integration Theory and Practice* (pp. 137-165). Philadelphia, PA: F.A. Davis.

Cheatum, B.A. & A. Hammond (1999). *Physical Activities for Improving Children's Learning and Behavior: A Guide to Sensory Motor Development.* Champaign, IL: Human Kinetics.

DeGangi, G.A. (1991). Assessment of sensory, emotional, and attentional problems in regulatory disordered infants: Part 2. In *Infants and Young Children,* 3(3), 9-19.

DeGangi, G.A. & R.A. Berk (1983). *DeGangi-Berk Test of Sensory Integration.* Los Angeles, CA: Western Psychological Services.

DeGangi, G.A. (2000). *Pediatric Disorders of Regulation and Affect in Behavior: A Therapist's Guide to Assessment and Treatment.* San Diego, CA: Academic Press.

Dunn, W. (1997). The impact of sensory processing abilities on the daily lives of young children and their families: A conceptual model. In *Infants and Young Children,* 9, 23-35.

Dunn, W. (1994). Performance of typical children on the sensory profile: An item analysis. *American Journal of Occupational Therapy, 48,* 967-974.

Dunn, W. (1991). The sensorimotor systems: A framework for assessment and intervention. In F.P. Orelove & D. Dobsey (Eds.), *Educating Children with Multiple Disabilities: A Transdisciplinary Approach* (2nd ed.). Baltimore, MD: Paul H. Brookes.

Dunn, W. (1999). *The Sensory Profile: User's Manual.* San Antonio, TX: Psychological Corporation.

Dunn, W., B.S. Myles & S. Orr. (2002). Sensory processing issues associated with Asperger syndrome: A preliminary investigation. *The American Journal of Occupational Therapy, 56,* 97-102.

Dunn, W., J. Saiter & L. Rinner. (2002). Asperger syndrome and sensory processing: A conceptual model and guidance for intervention planning. *Focus on Autism and Other Developmental Disabilities, 17*(3), 172-185.

Edelson, S.M., M.G. Edelson, D.C. Kerr & T. Grandin. (1999). Behavioral and physiologic effects of deep pressure on children with autism: A pilot study evaluating the efficacy of Grandin hug machine. *American Journal of Occupational Therapy, 53*(2) 145-52.

Fisher, A.G., E.A. Murray & A.C. Bundy (1991). *Sensory Integration Theory and Practice.* Philadelphia, PA: F.A. Davis.

Flowers, T. (1996). *Reaching the Child with Autism Through Art: Practical, Fun Activities to Enhance Sensory Motor Skills and to Improve Tactile and Concept Awareness.* Arlington, TX: Future Horizons.

Folio, M.R. & R.R. Fewell. (1983). *Peabody Developmental Motors: Scales and Activity Cards Manual.* Chicago, IL: Riverside.

Frick, S.M. (2001). *Listening With the Whole Body.* Madison, WI: Vital Links.

Frick, S, R. Frick, P. Oetter & E. Richter (1996). *Out of the Mouths of Babes: Discovering the Developmental Significance of the Mouth.* Hugo, MN: PDP Press, Inc.

Gardner, M.F. (1995). *Test of Visual-Motor Skills—Revised Manual.* Los Angeles, CA: Western Psychological Services.

Grandin, T. (1996). Brief report: Responses to national institutes of health report. *Journal of Autism and Developmental Disorders, 26* (2), 185-187.

Grandin, T. (1995). The learning style of people with autism: An autobiography. In K. Quill (Ed.), *Teaching Children with Autism: Strategies to Enhance Communication and Socialization* (pp.33-52). New York, NY: Delmar.

Grandin, T. "Teaching tips for children and adults with autism." *Center for the Study of Autism* (December 2002). Available online at www.autism.org/temple/tips.html.

Grandin, T. (1996). *Thinking in Pictures and Other Reports from My Life with Autism.* New York, NY: Vintage Books.

Greenspan, S. (1995). *The Challenging Child: Understanding, Raising, and Enjoying the Five "Difficult" Types of Children.* Reading, MA: Addison-Wesley.

Hanft, B. (2005). *Strategies for Students with Sensory Processing Disorders—Adapting School Environments.* Scientific Symposium on SPD: Bethesda, MD.

Hanft, B.E., L.J. Miller & S.J. Lane. (2000). Toward a consensus in terminology in sensory integration theory and practice: Part 3: Observable behaviors: Sensory integration dysfunction. *Sensory Integration Special Interest Section, 23* (3), 1-4.

Hannaford, C. (1995, revised 2005). *Smart Moves: Why Learning is Not All in Your Head.* Salt Lake City, UT : Great River Books.

Henderson, S.E. & D.A. Sugden. (1992). *Movement Assessment Battery for Children.* London: Psychological Corporation, Ltd.

Henry, D. (1998). *Tool Chest for Teachers, Parents & Students: A Handbook to Facilitate Self-Regulation.* Youngtown, AZ: Henry Occupational Therapy Services, Inc.

Howlin, P., L. Wing & J. Gould. (1995). The recognition of autism in children with Down syndrome: Implications for intervention and some speculations about pathology. *Developmental Medicine and Child Neurology, 37*(5), 406-414

Huebner, R.A. (2001). *Autism: A Sensorimotor Approach to Management.* Gaithersburg, MD: Aspen Publishers.

Huebner, R. & W. Dunn. (2001). "Introduction and basic concepts." In Huebner, R. (ed.), *Autism: A Sensorimotor Approach to Management* (pp. 3-36). Gaithersburg, MD: Aspen Publishers.

Kashman, N. & J. Mora. (2005). *The Sensory Connection.* Las Vegas, NV: Sensory Resources.

Kientz, M. & W. Dunn. (1997). A comparison of the performance of children with and without autism on the sensory profile. *American Journal of Occupational Therapy, 51*, 530-537.

Kimball, J.G. (1993). Sensory integrative frame of reference. In P. Kramer & J. Hinojosa (Eds.), *Frames of Reference for Pediatric Occupational Therapy* (pp. 87-169). Baltimore, MD: Williams & Wilkins.

Koomar, J. & A. Bundy. (1991). The art and science of creating direct intervention from theory. In A. Fisher, E. Murray, & A. Bundy (Eds.), *Sensory Integration Theory and Practice* (pp. 251-314). Philadelphia, PA: F.A. Davis.

Kranowitz, C.S. (1995). *101 Activities for Kids in Tight Spaces: At the Doctor's Office, On Car, Train, and Plane Trips, Home Sick in Bed....* New York, NY: St. Martin's Press.

Kranowitz, C.S. (2006). *Getting Kids in Sync: Sensory-Motor Activities to Help Children Develop Body Awareness and Integrate Their Senses.* Las Vegas, CA: Sensory Resources.

Kranowitz, C.S. (1998; revised 2006). *The Out-Of-Sync Child: Recognizing and Coping with Sensory Processing Disorder.* New York, NY: Perigee Books.

Kranowitz, C.S. (2003). *The Out-Of-Sync Child Has Fun—Activities for Kids with Sensory Integration Dysfunction.* New York, NY: Perigee Books.

Kranowitz, C., S. Szklut, L. Balzer-Martin, E. Haber & D. Sava. (2001). *Answers to Questions Teachers Ask About Sensory Integration.* Las Vegas. NV: Sensory Resources.

Lane, S. J., L.J. Miller & B.E. Hanft. (2000). Toward a consensus in terminology in sensory integration theory and practice: Part 2: Sensory integration patterns of function. *Sensory Integration Special Interest Section Quarterly, 23.*

Lashno, M. (1999). Sensory Integration: Observation of children with Down Syndrome and Autistic Spectrum Disorder. *Disability Solutions, 3*(5), 32-36.

Lester, B.M., K. Freier & L. La Gasse. (1995). Prenatal cocaine exposure and child outcome: What do we really know? In Lewis, M. & M. Bendersky (Eds.), *Mothers, Babies, and Cocaine: The Role of Toxins in Development* (pp. 19-40). Hillsdale, NJ: Erlbaum.

Lincoln, A.J., E. Courchesne, L. Harms & M. Allen. (1993). Contextual probability evaluation in autistic, receptive developmental language disorder: Event-related brain potential evidence. *Journal of Autism and Developmental Disorders, 23*(1), 37-57.

Lincoln, A.J., E. Courchesne, L. Harms & M. Allen. (1995). Sensory modulation of auditory stimuli in children with autism and receptive developmental language disorder: Event-related brain potential evidence. *Journal of Autism and Developmental Disorders, 25*(5), 521-539.

Lovass, I., C. Newson & C. Hickman. (1987). Self-stimulating behavior and perceptual reinforcement. *Journal of Applied Behavior Analysis, 20*(1): 45-68.

McClure, M.K. & M. Holtz-Yotz. (1991). The effects of sensory stimulatory treatment on an autistic child. *American Journal of Occupational Therapy, 45*(12), 1138-42.

McMullen. P. (2001). Living with sensory dysfunction in autism. In Huebner, R. (Ed)., *Autism: A Sensoriomotor Approach to Management* (pg. 472). Gaithersburg, MD: Aspen Publishers.

Mauro, T. & S. Cermak (2006). *The Everything Parent's Guide to Sensory Integration Disorder: Get the Right Diagnosis, Understand Treatments, and Advocate for Your Child.* Avon, MA: F&W Publications, Inc.

Miller, H. (1998). "Home activities for children with sensory integration problems." *SI Network—KID Foundation.*

Miller, L.J., S. Cermak, S. Lane, M. Anzalone & J. Koomar. (2004). Defining SPD and its subtypes—Position statement on terminology related to sensory integration dysfunction. *SI focus magazine, Summer 2004.*

Miller, L.J. & D. Fuller (2007). *Sensational Kids: Hope and Help for Children with Sensory Processing Disorder.* New York, NY: Perigee Trade.

Miller, L.J. & S.J. Lane. (2000). Toward a consensus in terminology in sensory integration theory and practice. Part 1—Taxonomy of neurophysiological processes. *Sensory Integration Special Interest Section Quarterly, 23*(1), 1-4.

Miller-Kuhaneck, H. (2004). *Autism: A Comprehensive Occupational Therapy Approach, 2nd Edition*. Bethesda, MD: AOTA Press.

Myers, B.A. & S.M. Pueschel. (1991). Psychiatric disorders in a population with Down syndrome. *Journal of Nervous and Mental Disorders, 179*, 609-613.

Nackley, V. (2001). Sensory diet applications and environmental modifications: A winning combination. *Sensory Integration Special Interest Section Quarterly, 24*(1), 1-4.

Ornitz, E.M. (1989). Autism at the interface between sensory and information processing. In G. Dawson (Ed.), *Autism: Nature, Diagnosis and Treatment*. New York, NY: Guilford.

Parham, D. & L. Fazio (Eds.). (1997). *Play in Occupational Therapy for Children*. St. Louis, MO: Mosby.

Reeves, G. (2001). "From neuron to behavior: Regulation, arousal and attention as important substrates for the process of sensory integration." In Smith-Roley, S., E. Imperatore-Blanche & R.C. Schaaf (Eds.), *The Nature of Sensory Integration with Diverse Populations*. San Diego, CA: Academic Press.

Reisman, J. (1993). Using a sensory integrative approach to treat self-injurious behaviour in an adult with profound mental retardation. *American Journal of Occupational Therapy, 47*(5) 403-410.

Reisman, J.E. & Hanschu, B. (1992). *Sensory Integration Inventory* (Rev. ed.). Hugo, MN: PDP Products.

Rodgers, S.J., S.L. Hepburn, T. Stackhouse & E. Wehner. (2003). Imitation performance in toddlers with autism and those with other developmental disorders. *Journal of Child Psychology and Psychiatry, 44*, 763-781.

Schaff, R.C. & M.E. Anzalone. (2001). Sensory integration with high-risk infants and young children. In Smith-Roley, S., E.I. Blanche & R.C. Schaaf (Eds.), *Sensory Integration with Diverse Populations*. (pp. 275-299). San Antonio, TX: Therapy Skill Builders.

Smith-Roley, S. (1999). *Course Manual: From Interpretation to Intervention: Course 3 of the Comprehensive Program in Sensory Integration*. Los Angeles, CA: Western Psychological Services.

Smith-Roley, S., E. Blanche & R. Schaaf (Eds). (2001). *Understanding the Nature of Sensory Integration with Diverse Populations*. San Antonio, TX: The Psychological Corporation.

Stehli, A. (1991). *The Sound of a Miracle: A Child's Triumph Over Autism*. New York, NY: Bantam Doubleday Dell Publishing Group.

Stern, D.N. (1985). *The Interpersonal World of the Infant*. New York, NY: Basic Books.

Tickle-Degnen, L. & W.J. Costner. (1995). Therapeutic interaction and the management of challenge during the beginning minutes of sensory integration treatment. *Occupational Therapy Journal of Research, 15*, 122-141.

Trott, M.C., M.K. Laurel & S.L. Windeck (1993). *SenseAbilities: Understanding Sensory Integration*. San Antonio, TX: The Psychological Corporation.

Wainwright-Sharp, J.A. & S.E. Bryson. (1993). Visual orienting deficits in high functioning people with autism. *Journal of Autism and Development Disorders, 23*(1), 1-13.

Waitling, R., J. Deitz, E. Kanny & J. McLaughlin. (1999). Current practice of occupational therapy for children with autism. *American Journal of Occupational Therapy 53*, 498-505.

Watling, R.L., J. Deitz & O. White. (2001). Comparison of sensory profile scores of young children with and without autism spectrum disorders. *American Journal of Occupational Therapy, 55*, 416-423.

Wilbarger, P. (1995). The sensory diet: Activity programs based on sensory processing theory. Sensory Integration Special Interest Section Newsletter, 18(2), 1-3.

Wilbarger, P. & J. Wilbarger. (1991). Sensory Defensiveness in Children Aged 2-12: An Intervention Guide for Parents and Other Caretakers. Santa Barbara, CA: Avanti Educational Programs.

Williams, D. (1944). *Somebody, Somewhere: Breaking Free From the World of Autism*. New York. NY: Times Books.

Williams, M. & S. Shellenberger. (1992). *An Introduction to "How Does Your Engine Run?" The Alert Program for Self-Regulation*. Albuquerque, NM: Therapy-Works.

Williams, M. & S. Shellenberger. (1996). *How Does Your Engine Run?: A Leader's Guide to the Alert Program for Self-Regulation*. Albuquerque, NM: Therapy Works, Inc.

Williams, M. & S. Shellenberger. (2001). *Take Five: Staying Alert at Home and School.* Albuquerque, NM: Therapy Works, Inc.

Williamson, G.G. & M.E. Anzalone (2001). *Sensory Integration and Self-Regulation in Infants and Toddlers: Helping Very Young Children Interact with their Environment.* Washington, D.C.: Zero to Three.

Worwood, V.A. (1991). *The Complete Book of Essential Oils and Aromatherapy: Over 600 Natural, Non-Toxic and Fragrant Recipes to Create Health & Beauty & a Safe Home Environment.* Novato, CA: New World Library.

Worwood, V.A. (1996). *The Fragrant Mind: Aromatherapy for Personality, Mind, Mood and Emotion.* Novato, CA: New World Library.

Resources

Throughout this book, many different types of toys, objects, and activities have been discussed or recommended for improving sensory processing disorder. Many items are simple everyday things that can be found around the home, easily made, or inexpensively purchased through catalogs, websites, and toy or dollar stores. Below are listed various sources for these items, as well as useful websites and organizations that can help you help your child with SPD.

Sensory Equipment and Toys

Below is a nonexhaustive list of objects that can be used with your child's sensory diet. Although some items are listed under a specific section, be aware that many provide benefits to other sensory systems as well. For example, playdough is good for tactile input as well as proprioceptive input.

Tactile

- Squeeze toys and fidgets with different textures (dog toys are actually the best and are relatively inexpensive)
- Playdough, Floam, Silly Putty, clay, Theraputty
- Koosh balls
- Foam puzzles

- Vibrating pens and balls (e.g., Bumble Ball)
- Velcro toys
- Shaving cream
- Pudding
- Wikki Stix
- Rubbery, sticky animals
- Beanbags
- Sand (Moon Sand is least messy)
- Stuffed animals
- Sensory box filled with beans, Styrofoam peanuts, small seashells, marbles, etc.
- Ribbons, yarn, fabric swatches
- Bubble wrap
- Finger and hand puppets
- Silly String
- Textured books and puzzles

Proprioceptive

- Balls, e.g., Nerf, Gertie, Koosh, vibrating
- Vibrating toys such as massagers, pens, Bumble Balls
- Squirt toys
- Paper punches
- Pop beads
- Wiggle cushions
- Weighted vests, blankets
- Beanbags
- Beanbag pillows (some also vibrate)
- Playdough press, cookie cutters
- Velcro mitt & ball
- Trampolines
- Ladders and climbing apparatus
- Body Sock
- DreamKuddle body pillow (provides deep pressure for sleeping)
- Tunnels, tents
- Bop bag
- Punch balls
- Ball pit
- Slinky

Vestibular

- Swings, sliding boards, gliders
- Large balls to sit, bounce, or roll on (Hippity Hop, Rody, Theraball)
- Sit 'n' Spin
- Hammock
- Trapeze
- Rocking chair
- Rocking horse
- Scooter
- Bicycle

Oral-Motor

- Whistles
- Straws (for blowing or sucking)
- Chewy tubes
- Nuk brushes
- Vibrating tooth brushes
- Bubbles (for blowing)
- Party horns, kazoos, harmonicas
- Pinwheels

Auditory

- Head phones (to reduce noise)
- Ear plugs
- Metronomes
- Percussion toys (e.g., tambourines, canastas, bongo drums)
- Rainsticks
- Keyboards
- Talking storybooks

Visual

- Flashlights
- Visual timers
- Light up squeeze toys

- Mylar paper and balloons
- Clear toys with small balls inside
- Lava lamps

Sensory Games and Activities

Below is a list of some games and activities that will help your child develop eye-hand coordination and improve motor coordination. The level of participation will depend on your child's motivation and how well he can follow directions.

- **Card games**, e.g., Go Fish, War, Old Maid, Uno
- **Memory games.** Many now are geared towards popular children's shows (Dora the Explorer, Sesame Street), which may help motivate your child to engage
- **Eye-Hand coordination games**, e.g., Hungry, Hungry Hippos, Hands Down, Topple, Simon, Perfection, Jenga
- **Motor Planning games**, e.g., Twister, Etch a Sketch
- **Fine Motor strength & dexterity games**, e.g., Legos, Duplos, Lincoln Logs, Tinker Toys, Coloring/Drawing, Playdough, Light Brite, Colorforms
- **Gross Motor games**, e.g., playground equipment, obstacle courses
- **Downloadable activities.** There are many websites available that offer free downloadable pages for educational, craft, and fine motor activities. Some favorites are listed below:
  - ❏ *www.activitypad.com* offers printable preschool activities, puzzles, learning games, and coloring pictures.
  - ❏ *www.do2learn.com* offers free teacher and parent materials, picture cards, educational games and art projects, daily organizers, and PECs products (some free and some to purchase).
  - ❏ *www.enchantedlearning.com* is available by subscription and has an excellent selection of educational-based printouts for preschool to elementary age children. Also provides simple craft activities for various age groups.

- *www.crayola.com* offers many theme-based crafts, coloring, and cutting projects. Also has separate information pages for parents, teachers, and websites for kids.
- *www.handwritingforkids.com* features printable worksheets for kids in preschool (shapes) to elementary school (manuscript and cursive). Also includes a section for "make your own" worksheets.
- *www.blackdog4kids.com* offers activities for preschoolers to teens, including puzzles, word searches, educational and holiday-oriented crafts, and printable and online games.
- *www.dltk-kids.com* offers printable pages of popular cartoon characters for coloring and themed craft activities. Includes projects for holidays.

Catalog Companies

The following catalogs are excellent sources for therapeutic toys and equipment. Keep in mind that an item you may see in a catalog may be found much cheaper at a discount store. For example, a soft squeezable toy dog that costs ten dollars in a catalog may also be available at your local dollar store.

Abilitations
www.abilitations.com
(800) 850-8602
Carries a lot of special needs equipment but also has a nice selection of sensory equipment, along with products for a multi-sensory room.

Achievement Products for Children
http://www.specialkidszone.com/
(800) 373-4699
Sells many products to meet the needs of children with special needs. Also carries an excellent selection of products to provide vestibular and proprioceptive input, along with a wide selection of oral motor tools.

Beyond Play
www.beyondplay.com
(877) 428-1244
Has a wide selection of toys including cause/effect toys, sensory toys, movement toys, ball pits, etc. Also has a large selection of books on autism, sensory issues, and fine motor skills.

In Your Pocket Designs
www.weightedvest.com
(888) 388-3224
Sells weighted vests and patterns for sewing your own. They also sell novelty weighted dress-up clothing.

Integrations
www.integrationscatalog.com
(800) 850-8602
This company is owned by Abilitations but the focus of this catalog is mostly on sensory toys. Also includes great tips about how a particular object will assist the sensory system (calming, organizing, etc.)

Jump-In Products
www.jump-in-products.com
(810) 231-9042
Therapist owned company featuring many Wilbarger brushing products. Has a nice selection of hand and oral motor toys.

Kidzplay/Theragifts
www.kidzplay.org
(603) 437-3330
Specializes in a variety of toys for children with sensory processing issues. Has a reasonably priced home suspension system for children needing vestibular input.

Learning Gear Plus
www.learninggearplus.com
(978) 597-9056
The majority of the products sold in this catalog are geared towards school/education but it also sells some adaptive equipment, such as pencil grippers.

Office Playground
www.officeplayground.com
(800) 458-1948
Has an excellent selection of fidgets and fine motor gadgets.
Reasonably priced.

Oriental Trading Company, Inc.
www.orientaltrading.com
(800) 875-8480
Offers a wide variety of inexpensive toys that can be used as
fidgets, as well as fine motor objects and craft kits.

PlayAway Toy Company
www.playawaytoy.com
(715) 752-4840
Sells a unique suspension system that can be hung in a door-
way for conducting therapy in the home. Reasonably priced.

Pocket Full of Therapy
www.pfot.com
(800) PFOT-124.
Well-known catalog to many therapists with a lot of sensory
toys to help with calming, organizing, and alerting a child's
sensory system. Catalog has a nice variety of therapeutic
games and activities.

Professional Development Programs (PDP Products)
www.pdppro.com
(877) 439-8865
Numerous sensory products and a nice selection of CDs for
listening and calming. Also has a good selection of books on
sensory processing for professionals and parents.

Really Good Stuff
www.reallygoodstuff.com
(800) 366-1920
Mostly educational products and a good selection of organizers, handwriting products, and educational charts.

Sensory Comfort
www.sensorycomfort.com
(888) 436-2622
Offers many products for children and adults with sensory issues, such as seam-free socks, cotton tank-top bras. Also headphones to decrease noise for children who are oversensitive to sound.

Sensory Tools
www.genjereb.com
(608) 819-0540
Offers a great selection of current books on sensory processing issues seen in different groups such as those with autism, AD/HD, and learning disabilities. Books are intended for many audiences, including professionals, parents, and children.

Southpaw Enterprises
www.southpawenterprises.com
(800) 228-1698
Very well-known catalog to many therapists. This is a large company that offers products for children with sensory integration/sensory processing difficulties, along with many products and books for children with various developmental concerns.

Sportime
www.sportime.com
(800) 283-5700
Features many items for physical activities, such as mats, tunnels, and obstacle courses.

Therapro
www.theraproducts.com
(800) 257-5376
Large company offering a vast selection of products for children with developmental delays or sensory processing issues. Sells a good selection of sensory stories, adaptive equipment for daily activities, and a selection of reusable daily checklists for children that have difficulty with organizing.

The Therapy Shoppe
www.therapyshoppe.com
(800) 261-5590
Therapist owned company with a wide selection of products, including specialty toys and games. Features a product called calming cards that teaches various calming strategies. Also has a good selection of chair cushions for children who need to move to help organize their sensory systems.

U.S. Games
www.us-games.com
(800) 327-0484
Equipment for movement and motor planning, including tunnels, cones, games, and objects for climbing, balance, and tossing.

Organizations

The following is a nonexhaustive list of organizations that provide information about sensory processing, parental support, advocacy, and treatment approaches.

American Occupational Therapy Association, Inc.
4720 Montgomery Lane
PO Box 31220
Bethesda, MD 20824-1220
(301) 652-2682
www.aota.org
Provides in-depth information about occupational therapy and may be able to help you locate sensory-experienced therapists within your area.

Occupational Therapy Systematic Evaluation of Evidence: OT Seeker
OTseeker Project Manager
Department of Occupational Therapy
The University of Queensland
Brisbane QLD 4072
Australia

www.otseeker.com
This site has a database that contains abstracts of systematic reviews and random controlled trials associated with OT research. The site has been developed in order to help consumers learn more information about the validity of certain types of treatment approaches. Also provides links to other sites with evidence-based practice.

SPD Network
5655 S. Yosemite St., Ste 305
Greenwood Village, CO 80111
(303) 794-1182
www.SPDnetwork.org
Provides information about SPD and includes resources for professionals and parents. Contains a directory of occupational, physical, and speech therapists that have a specific interest in SPD. Also contains a list of facilities and community resources available nationwide.

Wrightslaw Special Education Law and Advocacy
http://www.wrightslaw.com/
Site offers parents, educators, advocates, and attorneys accurate and reliable information about special education law, education law, and advocacy for children with special needs.

Yahoo
www.yahoogroups.com
Type in a search on "sensory processing" or "sensory dysfunction" and this will lead you to many other sites of interest concerning this topic.

Index